DEEP
LISTENING

DEEP LISTENING

A Healing Practice
to Calm Your Body,
Clear Your Mind, *and*
Open Your Heart

JILLIAN PRANSKY

with Jessica Wolf

RODALE.

RODALE *wellness*

Live happy. Be healthy. Get inspired.

Sign up today to get exclusive access to our authors, exclusive bonuses, and the most authoritative, useful, and cutting-edge information on health, wellness, fitness, and living your life to the fullest.

Visit us online at RodaleWellness.com
Join us at RodaleWellness.com/Join

Rodale books may be purchased for business or promotional use or for special sales. For information, please e-mail: BookMarketing@Rodale.com.

Printed in the United States of America

Rodale Inc. makes every effort to use acid-free ∞, recycled paper ♺.

Photographs by Mitch Mandel/Rodale Images

Book design by Carol Angstadt
Freelance designer: Ariana Abud

Library of Congress Cataloging-in-Publication Data is on file with the publisher.

ISBN 978–1–62336–856–2 hardcover

Distributed to the trade by Macmillan

2   4   6   8   10   9   7   5   3   1   hardcover

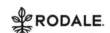

We inspire health, healing, happiness, and love in the world.
Starting with you.

FOR MY MOM AND DAD,
PHYLLIS, AND PAUL.
THANK YOU.

CONTENTS

Introduction 1

CHAPTER ONE
Welcome 10

CHAPTER TWO
Let Yourself Land 27

CHAPTER THREE
Being *Here* 49

CHAPTER FOUR
How We Hold 75

CHAPTER FIVE
Making Space 102

CHAPTER SIX
Listening Softly 128

CHAPTER SEVEN
Listening Deeply 152

CHAPTER EIGHT
Listening Bravely 180

CHAPTER NINE
Listening Again and Again and Again 208

CHAPTER TEN
A Deep Listening Practice:
   Putting It All Together 232

How to Prepare for Your Practice 263

Acknowledgments 268

Index 274

You are not a drop in the ocean.
You are the entire ocean in a drop.

—RUMI

INTRODUCTION

THE DEEP LISTENING JOURNEY

Deep Listening is the process of truly connecting to ourselves and our lives. It isn't so much a specific technique as it is an approach to how we receive and respond to ourselves and others.

Over the past 25 years, Deep Listening has helped me recover from injuries, illness, and grief. It has helped me better understand my challenging relationships and become closer to the people who are important to me. And through teaching this practice, I've discovered a number of things. Namely:

Most of us are used to living life as a series of reactions to what's going on around us.

Most of us feel stressed and overwhelmed much of the time.

Most of us live with tension in our body that is wreaking havoc on our health.

Most of us suffer from anxiety and don't know why it arises.

Most of us carry around powerful emotional narratives—the "stories" we tell ourselves about our undigested pain—and we're not sure how to heal those hurts from the past.

Most of us don't understand how to change the habits that keep us stuck.

And most of us don't know how to be gentle, kind, and compassionate with ourselves—the conditions that allow us to evolve.

The more I've learned about how our bodies work, how our minds work, and how *stress* is at the root of so much of our fatigue, burnout, anxiety, addiction, and illness, the more I've been able to organically incorporate that information into my teaching.

But the truth is, stress is not really the problem. The problem is that we need to *respond* differently—not only to stress but to anything that makes us uncomfortable. And most of us have no idea how to do that.

Deep Listening is the habit of paying close and tender attention to our body, our mind, and our heart so we can meet our "stress" differently. This type of attention provides us with more resources and a greater capacity—physically, mentally, emotionally, and relationally—to respond calmly, clearly, and wisely, and also to engage more fully and expansively in our life.

We're going to develop Deep Listening tools that focus on *experiencing* our connectedness. This feeling of connection not only changes the way we respond to stress, it actually leaves us feeling less stressed, increases the amount of joy in our life, and sets the conditions for us to evolve.

That might sound like a big promise, but it's not. We're *designed* to feel deep connections. And we are going to learn how.

The Arc of Our Journey

Slowly and gently, we are going to develop a strong foundation that we can rest on any and every time we meet challenges in life.

After each chapter, you'll find a short series of practices to bring the material to life. I highly recommend trying at least a few as you move through the book. They offer a deeper understanding of the material and help us recognize all that we hold in our body and mind—and, of course, how to release it. But more important, the practices offer us a deeper understanding of ourselves.

To begin, we're going to focus on our body and mind, exploring, little by little, the limitations that keep us from experiencing our own well-being. Later on, we'll go deeper, using what we've learned to develop a practice that sets the conditions to live more openheartedly.

This work is sequential and progressive—meaning the techniques we practice early on allow us to develop the practices that come later. But the material is also interconnected. So while each practice technique can be done on its own, it's the sum of the practices that creates the framework for us to become more calm, clear, and open. As you'll see: Everything you do adds up.

A Little + Often = A Lot

If you're new to a daily practice, the idea of doing something every day may seem daunting. But I encourage my students to do a little bit often rather than feel they have to take on a lot all at once. I've always believed that we get the best results when we work at a pace that feels right for us *personally*. However, my faith in how much benefit we get from small, quiet changes was solidified a few years ago through an experience I had with my son, William.

William was born with a life-threatening allergy to gluten and wheat. That means that if he ate a pretzel handed to him by a well-meaning toddler, he would stop breathing. When you have to guard your child from almost everything his friends are likely to be eating, it's pretty terrifying. Then, when you start imagining your child away at college, having a few drinks and accidently taking a bite of a hamburger, you become completely overwhelmed.

William was so allergic that he would have an anaphylactic reaction if he were merely kissed by someone who had traces of wheat on their lips. In fact, the severity of his allergies was one of the reasons we were invited to participate in a clinical study about building tolerance to wheat.

Every other week for 2 years, William was given microscopic amounts of wheat in progressively larger doses. He started with 6 milligrams—just shy of the amount that would trigger his anaphylaxis. For context, a teaspoon of wheat is about 2,700 milligrams.

Over the course of the study, my son went from being unable to tolerate a wheat-on-the-lips kiss to being able to eat a slice of bread with no reaction.

Milligram by milligram, William grew more resilient. This was life-changing for him.

We can *all* change our lives this way—slowly and gently, in tiny increments.

Our Deep Listening Toolbox

The tools we'll use are simple and may even be familiar to you—meditation, yoga, relaxation, mindfulness, journaling, and an "Instant Pause and Reset" technique that can be done anywhere, at any time.

These mind-body practices are designed to balance the nervous system and have been known to increase immune function, enhance the process of digestion, and set the whole body up for deep healing, growth, and repair. They also help us discover and release the tension we hold, making us more comfortable and at ease in our body. Some people report having more energy. Some say they sleep better. My students tell me they see big differences in their health, their relationships, and the choices they make day to day. These tools help us develop the skills that, over time, can actually transform our lives.

You can build your practice in your own time and based on your own interest and needs. Some people gravitate toward one single technique, such as the yoga poses. Others explore all the techniques offered in each practice section. You can work with these practices in whatever way suits you.

Taking a slow, gentle approach to your body, your mind, and your life may feel awkward at first. This may not be something you are used to, so it may require a small leap of faith on your part to believe that it will all be worthwhile.

It will.

Remember: A little + often = a lot.

About the Practices

The Yoga Experiences in this book are not designed as workouts. As you'll see, we're going to move away from an "achieving" mentality, so the point of the practices is not to get them "right" but rather to have an "experience." Each movement is an opportunity to practice paying attention to your body in an open and nourishing way. If your ability to move is limited or your doctor does not recommend certain movements, please modify the exercises so they are appropriate for you.

I recommend reading the instructions all the way through before you begin each pose. The first few moments in a pose may feel awkward; this is normal. Take a few breaths and adjust your body, giving yourself time to feel more natural. Continue to make any micro-adjustments as you need throughout your time in a pose.

The Meditation Experiences and the Restorative Yoga Experiences can be done on their own or before or after yoga. I recommend reading the instructions all the way through before you begin.

You can do the meditations lying down, seated on the ground, or in a chair. I usually practice in a private, quiet space, but I've practiced meditation everywhere: on the train, at my desk, sitting in my parked car, in the doctor's office, and even in the bathroom at family gatherings. I often set a timer for the duration I'd like to practice. Visit page 263 for guidance on preparing a meditation seat.

Once you set up the restorative yoga experience, you may want to spend 5 to 15 minutes relaxing into the pose. For a *guided* relaxation, slowly recite the *Relaxmore* section into a voice recorder and listen to it during your practice. The *Relaxmore* offers cues to release stress and tension and also allows you to more deeply absorb the teachings. Visit page 263 for guidance on preparing your props for restorative yoga.

To support your practice, I have made recordings of the meditations I offer in this book. You can find them at jillianpransky.com/deeplisteningmeditations.

In either experience, feel free to make adjustments anytime you need to feel more comfortable.

We practice on the mat

so our skills become

second nature

in the face of stress.

The Contemplations and **Journaling Prompts** allow us to hear our quiet, inner voice. This voice is the seed from which long-term change becomes possible. Both practices help integrate the benefits from all our other exercises.

I recommend getting a notebook that you can devote to your journaling. Although I've kept a diary since I was 9 (my first one had a Snoopy cover), many of my students have never written a single journal entry. You do not need to be a "writer" to journal!

Please don't spend time worrying about what you "should" write. If my prompts don't resonate with you, I invite you to make up your own.

The Instant Pause and Resets allow you to quickly refresh and shift your energy. They have been one of my most treasured tools for getting calm and clear.

Let me tell you a secret: Even after more than two decades of yoga and meditation practice, I still need help centering myself when something sends me reeling. So I created these short, three-breath "resets" that I use throughout the day.

Here's another secret: I don't wait until I need them. I usually schedule them into my routine, maybe three times a day. In fact, on days when I know really need the extra support, I set my phone alarm every 2 hours to remind me to Pause and Reset.

About Props and Equipment

Aside from a yoga mat, you may want to acquire or have a few other props on hand for the practices. I use props for support during yoga, comfort during relaxation, or to sit on during meditation. See page 263 for illustrations and instructions on how to prepare and use these props.

- **Two yoga blocks.** These are a worthwhile investment.
- **Four yoga blankets.** If you don't have yoga blankets, beach

towels will do. In some poses, large king-size bed pillows can work.

- **Yoga strap.** A belt or a long scarf will work, too.

Sample Weekly Practice Schedule

If you'd like to create a weekly practice, here's my suggestion for a place to start. You can do all of them, or pick and choose the practices that speak to you.

- **Yoga:** 5 to 60 minutes, four times per week
- **Restorative yoga:** 5 to 20 minutes, four times per week
- **Meditation:** 5 to 20 minutes daily
- **Instant Pause and Reset:** three times daily
- **Contemplation and/or journaling:** once per week

CHAPTER ONE

Welcome

When we feel welcomed,
we show up more.

My First Panic Attack

I'd been teaching yoga for almost 6 years when I had my first panic attack. My 34-year-old sister-in-law, Lisa, had died recently, and I'd gone to Maryland to help pack up her things. On the drive home to Hoboken, New Jersey, my arms went numb. I became dizzy and short of breath, my vision blurred, and my muscles were shaky and weak. I was sure I was having a heart attack. When I showed up at the hospital and the ER doctors diagnosed me with an anxiety attack, I argued with them. How could I be having an anxiety attack? I'm a yoga teacher.

When Lisa was 30 years old, she was diagnosed with asbestos-induced lung cancer. She was my oldest brother's wife, and even more significant than our closeness was that she was *like* me. This marked the first time someone I loved who was also *my own age* became seriously ill.

We were both young, active professional women at the beginning of our careers, eagerly stepping into adulthood. She was a step or two ahead of me, with a husband and a baby, but otherwise her circumstances could have been mine. Like Lisa, I had an abundance of spirit and ambition—and, I assumed, plenty of time to grow into a successful life. These realizations began as small thoughts when she was diagnosed, bouncing around inside me for all the years of her illness.

In boxing up Lisa's things—her well-worn cowboy boots, her Levi's jean jacket, her Mickey Mouse sweatshirt—a major truth began taking root inside me: We are not really in control of our life.

I had been no stranger to family illness. My father was in the hospital regularly throughout my life with heart disease, cancers, and kidney disease. But as a family, we focused our attention on doctor appointments and home care. We never talked about how we felt or how his illness was affecting us *inside*. If I cried about my father, it was alone in my room.

Initially, I dealt with Lisa's illness and death the same way: muscling through and pushing away my emotions. But my anxiety attack cracked my protective armor and revealed layers of vulnerability I had never experienced before. Suddenly, I could no longer muscle my way through anything. I felt afraid most of the time, and because I was in a constant state of anxiety, I began to see the world through a lens of fear. I was scared to ride the subway, scared to fly in a plane. Daily challenges that I used to conquer enthusiastically now made me shaky. I felt as if I were forever running away from danger.

When a major event, transition, or unexpected incident triggers a big shift in perspective, feelings we have buried for years often rise up, seemingly out of nowhere.

I now know that my panic attack was simply my first acute response to fears that I'd been living with my whole life but that only began to rise to the surface as I watched my sister-in-law's struggle. Fear about all the ways I was not enough: not strong enough to overcome illness, not talented enough to be successful in my job, not worthy enough to be loved.

I had turned to yoga in the past to get through difficult life events, but the fear I experienced around Lisa's death was different. And it launched the beginning of my deepest practice.

My Early Yoga

The first time I ever did yoga or meditation I was 9 years old. My mother had my brothers and me learn Transcendental Meditation, and she took me with her to yoga classes at the gym. She considered all of this "family therapy."

I was the only one in the family who enjoyed it, but I was passionate about most things. I was a go-getter from the get-go. I became president of every club I joined. I was a dedicated athlete. Over time, I grew into a "you-can-do-it" fitness instructor and an energetic young executive.

When Lisa became ill, I had (and taught) a yoga practice that was physical and athletic, like me. I'd built my entire identity around being able to achieve things. I loved how powerful my body felt when I practiced yoga. I loved the sensations of openness and expansiveness when challenging my physical boundaries. I did headstands so I could feel mighty and successful and strong.

In the wake of Lisa's death, I suffered from both anxiety and exhaustion. As my health faltered, I realized that the yoga practice I had created to make myself feel solid and secure was not the type of practice I needed to become a more active participant in my own well-being. It seems like someone who is the president of everything would be plenty active already, right? But I discovered that the many things I was actively pursuing all the time often did not support my health. I spent a lot of time *doing* and very little time *being*.

What Is Well-Being?

I think of *well-being* as the ability to live in a state of contentment. Contentment is a bit different from simply being happy. We usually think of happiness as dependent on a set of circumstances. Contentment, on the other hand, is not dependent on anything. It's a sense of not needing or wanting things to be different in order to feel "okay."

When we cultivate a sense of well-being, we are developing a relationship with ourselves that provides exactly the type of strength and security I thought I would find in mastering headstands.

Well-being is the ability to stay grounded, relaxed, and open to *whatever* your circumstances are. It's the freedom to be present with *whatever* is going on inside or outside of you. It's no longer suffering

—

from the exhaustion or disappointment of trying to make everything "just right." Spiritual teachers refer to this condition as the state of *equanimity*—being open to things just the way they are.

Well-being is available to anyone at any time. But, like headstands, it takes practice.

BE HERE, DO LESS

You don't need to travel to India to find contentment. You don't need to push yourself to "be better" or "do more" to have a sense of well-being. In fact, I invite my students to "be here" and "do less."

We cultivate well-being by *relaxing into the life that we have right now.* The notion that we can live better by striving less may seem like a radical concept in this age of relentless Internet searches and the endless barrage of information that's thrust toward us every day. It's certainly not the type of solution we're used to.

Fostering a sense of well-being does not require anything especially difficult. But it does require showing up and spending time with ourselves in a way we may not be accustomed to.

LET'S PAUSE FOR A MOMENT

Showing up starts with a simple action: We pause.

Pausing is an activity that's accomplished exactly the way

you'd think—we just stop for a bit. It's a small break that we take, on purpose, to gather ourselves.

When we pause, we take a moment to be with ourselves, right here, right now, in *whatever* state we're in. We don't have to do anything. We don't have to feel any particular way.

Pausing gives us extra room to take things in. It allows us time to listen to ourselves before responding or reacting. We pause so we can pay attention to ourselves, to others, and to the world around us in a more open and compassionate way. It's one of the main tools we use to release tension in our bodies and in our minds. It's one of the most valuable skills we can develop to change habits that do not serve us.

We are going to pause a lot together through this journey. I consider it my go-to tool. Pausing is not only a useful skill for day-to-day living, but, as we'll discover, it's also an always-available activity that we can use to transform our life.

WELCOME YOURSELF

E very time I practice, the first thing I do is pause and welcome myself.

Imagine for a moment what it's like to show up somewhere and feel welcome—really, really welcome. Imagine that moment when you truly sense how *delighted* someone is that you've arrived.

When we feel welcomed, we show up more.

There is no more powerful message we can send to ourselves than greeting ourselves with open arms.

Welcome

In whatever way you're showing up here . . .
wherever you may have been . . .
gather your whole self up
and let yourself know you're welcome here.

Whether you're showing up with expectations . . . or with fears . . .
whether you're showing up in joy . . . or in sorrow . . .
take a moment to greet yourself
exactly as you are right now.

Gather yourself up and welcome *all* of you:
your mind, your body, your breath.
Sit for a moment and welcome yourself
along with each breath as it fills you.

Welcome your breath into your body.
Welcome your mind onto your breath.
Welcome your body into the room.

Your breath is *always* welcoming you.

Meet your breath with your body.
Greet your breath with your body.
Take a moment to *be* with your breath.
Take a moment to *be* with yourself.

When we feel *welcomed*, we show up *more*.

—

Practices for Welcoming Ourselves

We are learning to welcome our breath into our body.
We are learning to welcome our mind onto our breath.
We are learning to create a safe space for ourselves,
so we can show up more.

CONTEMPLATION

Imagine being greeted by someone who would welcome you with great warmth. This could be a friend, family member, mentor, a spiritual teacher, or even a pet—anyone who you can imagine welcoming you wholeheartedly. If you had a video of this reception, what do you look like?

> *What would your posture be like?*
>
> *What would the expression on your face be as you were greeted?*
>
> *What does it feel like to be you, when you feel safe and welcomed?*

MEDITATION EXPERIENCE:
ELEVATOR TO A WELCOMING ARRIVAL

This simple technique uses visualization to help you feel more welcomed and safe.

- Sit in a comfortable position on the ground or in a chair. Close your eyes, if you wish. Take a few long exhales. Notice where your body meets support.
- Envision your body as a three-story building. Now imagine an elevator inside this building. The third floor is from your crown to your shoulders. The second floor is from your shoulders to your belly. The first floor is from your belly to where your seat meets support.
- Now imagine the elevator lowering down through the center of you one flight at a time.
- Begin at the crown of your head.
- Exhale: Envision the elevator lowering from crown to shoulders. Inhale: Imagine the doors of the elevator opening, fresh air and light coming in.
- Exhale: Let your weight drain down another flight, from shoulders to belly. Feel your inhale freshen you.
- Exhale: Continue to the ground floor. Allow your body weight to lower completely into your seat and legs. The elevator doors open on your inhale, filling you with reviving breath.
- Repeat this lowering process one to three more times.
- On your last elevator exhale, allow yourself to land completely

on the ground. And when the elevator doors open, imagine a dear one is there to greet you sweetly.

- Let this imagery fade and place one hand on your heart and one on your belly. Feel your breath under your hands. Stay with the feeling of your breath in your hands for a moment.

Welcome your breath with your hands.
Welcome your breath into your body.
Welcome your mind onto your breath, into your body.
Welcome yourself here, now, as you are.

- Sit for a few minutes longer, feeling yourself grounded, as you continually welcome your breath and yourself.
- To close, welcome yourself again into your seat, on the ground. Set an intention to stay with yourself as you transition out of the meditation.

You will repeatedly be pulled away from your

breath by thoughts, sensations, or sounds.

This is not a problem but a chance to

welcome yourself back,

to return to greet your breath,

over and over again, into the moment.

—

Yoga Experience: Hero Pose

PROPS: Two yoga blocks stacked. If needed, stack three blocks or sit on a chair and begin with the second bulleted step.

- Kneel, with your seat resting on your stacked blocks. Your inner thighs a few inches apart. The tops of your feet face-down along the sides of your block.
- With your hands, draw the muscular part of your back thighs out to the sides to more easily feel your sit bones on the support.
- Imagine the way an elevator lowers, one flight at a time, and gently lengthen your next three exhales as the elevator lowers from your head down to your shoulders, from your shoulders down to belly, and from your belly down to your seat and legs.
- Sit for 5 to 10 breaths, as you allow your blocks to hold you up completely.
- For the last few breaths, place your hands on your belly; feel your breath move under your hands. Welcome your breath into your hands. Welcome yourself onto the ground.
- Mindfully transition out of the pose when you are ready.

When you allow the ground to hold you,

you can release resistance,

you can release the tension

that would limit the flow of the breath.

When you feel more welcomed on the

ground, your breath is more welcome in you.

—

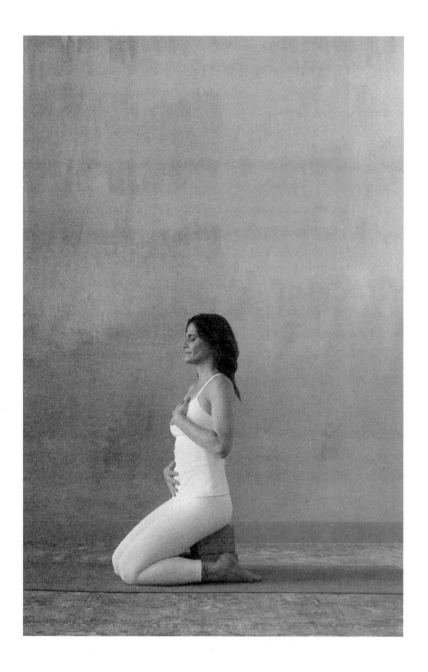

Restorative Yoga Experience: Constructive Rest

PROPS: Two long rectangle—folded blankets, stacked.

SET UP

- Lie down on your back, knees bent, feet on the floor, arms resting alongside your body. Bring your feet a few inches from your seat and a little wider apart than your hips.
- Let your knees fall together to hold each other up.
- Place your stack of blankets over your knees with the long ends draping down the sides of your legs. This will help you release all muscular effort in your legs.
- As you explore being in your yoga poses and restoratives, feel free to readjust with any micro movements that help you feel more comfortable, grounded, and at ease.

EXPERIENCE CONSTRUCTIVE REST

- Enjoy several long exhales as you progressively release your body weight into the ground. Allow your feet, seat, back, and head to fall into the embrace of the earth.
- Mindfully scan your face and soften any obvious squinting and clinching in the eyes, ears, and mouth. Let your tongue rest fully on the floor of your mouth.
- *Relaxmore* for 5 to 10 minutes.
- To prepare to finish, bring your hands to your belly and pause to feel your palms receiving your breath. Imagine the breath unraveling any lingering knots inside.

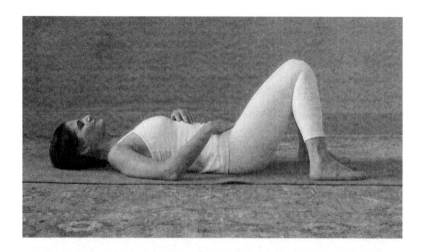

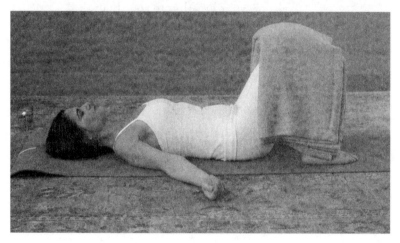

- Slowly transition out of the pose by taking the blankets off your legs and hugging both knees to your belly. Gently move in any way that feels good to you. Mindfully roll to your side and pause, then caringly press up to sitting.
- *Relaxmore* for 5 to 10 minutes.

Relaxmore
SHOW UP AND RELAX MORE

Let your feet land heavily on the ground.
Feel your footprints dropping deeper and deeper into the earth.
Effortless legs.
Your pelvis cradled by the earth.
Your back melts into the ground.
Feel the ground welcoming your shoulders and upper back,
Allow the earth to receive your head completely.

Welcome your breath into your body.
Welcome your breath with a softening belly.
Your breath caring for you as it flows in and out on its own.
Let your belly soften more and drain down into your back.

Let your body rest on the ground.
The earth will hold you.
Let your breath into your body.
The ground longs to carry you,
so your breath can fill you.

We are taught to hold in our belly.

When we soften our belly,

we can relax more deeply

and feel more welcome in our own bodies.

—

Journaling Prompt:
Invite Your Authentic Self

Can you welcome yourself here, just as you are?
Write an invitation or welcome note to yourself.

- Welcome yourself just as you are, right now, to this moment, to begin this Deep Listening practice you are embarking on.
- Invite yourself to participate as fully as you possibly can.
- Encourage yourself to keep an open mind and heart; to remain curious and present with all that unfolds, whether it be a delight or challenge.

Right now, can you make an unconditional
relationship with yourself?
Just at the height you are,
the weight you are,
with the current intelligence level you have,
with your current burden of pain.
Can you enter into an unconditional
relationship with that?
—Pema Chödrön

INSTANT PAUSE AND RESET:
A WARM GREETING

Use the welcoming elevator imagery for three breaths while you are in line at the grocery story, waiting at a red light, or even in a real elevator! Keep your eyes open as you turn your attention to your body and breath.

- Imagining the way an elevator lowers one flight at a time, use your next three exhales to lower your weight down from your head to your shoulders, from shoulders to belly, and finally from belly down into your seat, legs, and feet.
- Pause at the end of your third exhale and let yourself land fully.
- On your next inhale, envision your elevator doors opening and that a dear one is there to warmly greet you. Let yourself be received. Notice how you feel.
- To finish, welcome yourself into this moment, now, as you are.

CHAPTER TWO

Let Yourself Land

In order to feel "okay,"
we need to feel safe.
And in order to feel safe,
we need to feel stable and grounded.

I WAS ALWAYS DOING THINGS, ALL THE TIME

I grew up in a family of boys, where I felt that in order to be seen and to get approval, I had to succeed in measurable ways. I felt as though I always had to be getting better: better grades, better job, better position on the team. I wasn't enough just being me in the world.

As a young woman, I wanted to feel valuable, and I always felt valued when I worked. So I worked *more*. More jobs. More assignments. Better titles.

At 23, I decided to start running. I ran my first 5-mile race having never run 5 miles before in my life. Immediately afterward, someone said to me, "You should run a marathon." So 5 months later, my boss happened to have an extra spot in the New York City

Marathon, and, in a moment of misplaced enthusiasm, I took it.

Because I had cultivated a mind-over-matter attitude, I was actually able to cross the finish line. But then I was sick for a year. I had pushed myself too much, although I didn't make that connection at the time.

As a young mother, I had a baby with health issues, and I didn't sleep through the night for years. When my son was 3, I ended up having seizures that no one could determine the cause of. It didn't occur to me (or to my doctors) that I'd become ill from no longer being able to truly rest.

I loved my job. I loved my strong body. I loved being a mother. And because I was "good" at it all, I thought I was supposed to do *more* of it.

During each of my three health crises—a year-long bout with chronic fatigue following the marathon, panic attacks after Lisa died, and a complete physical breakdown after going years without enough sleep—I felt as if the ground had crumbled beneath me. I was a strong, can-do person—and then, suddenly, I wasn't.

I now have reverence for my burnout, my anxiety, and the way that I dropped completely. These trials were my teachers, forcing me to ask, "Why am I always pushing so hard?"

We Are Zippers

My favorite description of how hard we're always working comes from *True Refuge* by psychologist and meditation teacher Tara Brach.* She says, "It's like we're in a motorboat noisily zipping around, trying to find a place that is quiet, peaceful, and still. We're solving a problem, responding to demands, preparing for what's next, improving ourselves. But we're just making more waves and noise wherever we go. It counters all our ambitious conditioning, but true freedom comes when we throttle back the motor and come naturally to stillness."

We've become a society of *zippers*. Whether it's our endless to-do list or our feeling that we have to "get it right," we feel pushed and pulled all the time. For most of our lives, we've gotten the message that we have to get ahead—from our parents, from our teachers, and from the media. Even when most of us "try" to relax, we go about it in a zealous, goal-oriented way. I am as guilty of this as anyone. When I first discovered yoga, I felt the need to take classes 7 days a week for 3 years, then sign up for a teacher training. All my efforts at relaxation used to be about *getting better*.

Somehow, we believe that if we stop working so hard, something will not be *okay*. *We* will not be okay. And this creates a lot of stress.

When we're zipping around, it's as if we're forever running toward something or running away from something. And our nervous system thinks, "Oh, if you're running, things must not be okay. I'll help! I'll give you more of what you need to run!" And that "help" sets off a whole series of events in our body and in our mind.

When we are forever focused on overefforting, and overstriving, our nervous system is saying, "I better make sure we can conquer or get away."

—

29

What's Going On in Our Mind
When We're Zipping

The part of our brain that jumps in to help when we're zipping was designed, historically, to keep us safe. It's triggered *whenever* we feel threatened. In fact, this part of our brain—our fear center—even interprets *not feeling okay* as a type of a threat.

When we don't feel safe, our neurology shifts into survival mode.

Our higher-order, prefrontal cortex thinking goes offline and we lose access to our creative problem-solving abilities. Instead, we think and act from habit, past experience, or instinct.

Simultaneously, our brain releases the hormones we need to respond to danger—adrenaline, epinephrine, and cortisol. These chemicals provide us with the strength and energy we need to fight, flee, or freeze.

Our "stress hormones" not only get our body ready to act, they affect how we feel emotionally, and this "stress" manifests differently in each of us. Some of us lose our temper more easily. Others become anxious, always worrying that things are just not right. Some of us get depressed or cranky, or feel like the world is against us; others feel alone or misunderstood.

In any case, this hormone dump can leave us with a sense of restlessness that, for many of us, is so uncomfortable that we unconsciously spend much of our time and energy simply trying to make it go away. We might distract ourselves by eating when we're not hungry or shopping when we don't need things. We try to quell those unsettling feelings with alcohol or drugs or cigarettes or sex. Or we spend all our time working or exercising or making sure we're very, very busy.

The stress response leaves us ungrounded, so we become naturally and powerfully drawn to anything that makes us feel better quickly, even if it doesn't last.

So when we don't think we're "okay"—whether it's because we are white-knuckling during a turbulent flight, sweating through a job interview, or scrambling for our lost car keys—our brain is operating in emergency mode and we are *physiologically* unable to make considered and compassionate choices. We *react* rather than *respond*, and our reactions are informed by our survival instincts. We become hostile (fight), we run away from problems (flight), or we go numb (freeze). Because, as far as our neurology is concerned, we're in the face of a threat, and all that matters is that we get safe and things become *okay*. This is our biology—it's true for *all of us*.

We all want to feel centered and safe.

Yet the ways we're trying to get there

are actually creating more stress.

WHAT'S GOING ON IN OUR BODY

We usually regard stress as something that happens only in our mind. But when our survival mode is triggered, the systems in our body also shift.

—

Imagine our body is like a house and each room is a different physiological system. Several rooms are dedicated to long-term health and healing, and one big room is devoted specifically to our immediate survival. Energy is directed to these various rooms the way electricity might be distributed throughout a home.

Our long-term health and healing rooms are the ones primarily devoted to our longevity and overall wellness. So we have our Digestion Room, our Reproduction Room, our Immunity Room, our Elimination Room, and our Growth and Repair Room. When we are relaxed and calm, electricity flows easily to all those rooms.

However, when we feel unsafe, our brain instantly shuts down the flow of energy to those long-term health and healing rooms and instead sends all our energy straight to the Immediate Survival Room.

This house metaphor is a very simplistic way to understand the relationship between the stress response and the relaxation response—the dual aspects of our neurology that are in charge of either keeping us safe *or* keeping us nourished and well. Like a light switch that is either on or off, both of these responses cannot be engaged at the same time.

THE MIND-BODY CONNECTION

Most of us think of "feeling grounded" as a state of mind. However, the relationship between our mind and our body is so fundamental and interconnected that it almost makes no sense to discuss the two as separate entities. When we start to experience this connection, it allows us to understand how we can support ourselves emotionally by working with our body, and how we can support our physical healing by attending to our emotions.

So, *feeling grounded* does not necessarily occur only when we've cultivated a "balanced" mental state. It can also develop from noticing what it feels like when our body is completely supported by the earth.

OUR RELATIONSHIP WITH THE GROUND

As we grow up, we tend to forget what it's like to have a relationship with the ground. Think of how babies learn to roll from their backs to their bellies. They teach themselves slowly and deliberately to move in *relationship* with the ground. They press and push and *partner* with the ground to get the support they need to grow and thrive.

We are training to become more and more familiar with the moment when we feel ourselves—physically and emotionally—land on the ground. That moment when we exhale and we feel like we don't have to keep it all together and hold it all up and get it all done. We're training ourselves to notice that moment when we feel completely unencumbered, even for a very short time. The truth is, it calms our nervous system when we feel a sense of support in our life and in our world. Feeling separate or isolated can *create* stress. We need to learn how to experience our relatedness more than we're used to.

—

THE MIND-BODY *CONVERSATION*

Since one of the most powerful ways to feel more *okay* mentally and emotionally is to learn how to relax the body, we begin by learning how to release one of the most chronically tensed muscles in all of us.

The psoas is a long muscle that connects our legs to our spine. When we feel unsafe, this muscle contracts. In fact, it's the very first muscle that's activated if we need to fight, flee, or freeze. Think of a sprinter at the starting line of a race, ready to take off. That is the stance of a contracted psoas.

All day long, our nervous system is communicating with our psoas, and our psoas is sending information back to our nervous system. Imagine hiking in the woods and suddenly coming upon a snake. Most of us would be startled, and our fear center would immediately fire up our psoas to move us to safety. Similarly, if we're hiking a rocky trail and it's hard to keep our footing, that experience of being off balance is perceived by this muscle, and it not only engages to stabilize us, it also instantly sends our brain a signal that we're on dangerous ground. Mind and body are in constant conversation about our feelings of safety.

This communication system gets complicated when our daily habits affect messages to and from our psoas. For instance, the psoas contracts not only when we feel threatened but also when we drive, when we sit for too long, and when we walk on concrete. Even walking in certain shoes can tighten our psoas. In other words, this muscle becomes constricted from things most of us do every single day.

A tight psoas can cause back pain. Or, because it attaches in our midsection, a tight psoas can hamper digestion. As extreme as it sounds, this muscle can affect so many of our systems that when it's chronically constricted, not only can it leave us physically uncomfortable but it can also leave us emotionally unsettled and anxious.

When our psoas is tight, it's hard to sense ourselves landing on the ground. But when the psoas is malleable and pliable, it allows us to feel safe and grounded—like we *belong* on the earth.

The Practices for Landing on the Ground following this section are designed to leave us feeling more grounded as they help release excess holding in the psoas. I've also included a Supple Psoas Sequence in the Extended Practice Section on page 262.

When we don't feel "okay," the psoas gets tight.

And when the psoas is tight

it perpetuates the belief that we're not okay.

THE BENEFITS OF GROUNDING

When the psoas muscle can release, we can begin to experience that the ground is there to hold us. That it *will* hold us.

Once we feel the safety offered by the ground, we can begin to relax. Instead of our tendency to keep zipping around, trying to make things better, we can pause and listen to what is actually going on in our body and in our life. Because as we'll learn, when we view our life through a lens of stress, we often don't see things as they really are.

Experiencing life from a place of calmness and clarity changes us.

When we're calm, our brain turns our big-picture, prefrontal cortex thinking back on and we naturally begin making decisions that better serve us. We are able to listen confidently to our intuition, and our choices begin to emerge from deep wisdom and compassion.

If we want to operate from this place of calm, we need to throw back the throttle of our zipping boat and grow idle. The more we can feel in our mind *and* in our body that we are okay in the world being who we are—just being who we *already* are—the more we are able to experience feeling safe and at ease. And the more we can be at ease, the greater our sense of overall well-being.

When we learn to be supported by the ground,

we are able to live in a completely different way.

We are able to become more available to

ourselves and the people we love.

Landing

Slowly slide your mind through your body
and notice where your body meets the ground.
On each out breath
let your weight drop down
into the ground.

Let the earth hold you.
No need to grip.
No need to clench.
No need to prop yourself up
anywhere.

Let your body land on the ground.
Let your breath fill your body.
The ground holds you
so your breath can fill you.
Feel the earth holding you.

Let your body land completely.
Nothing to do. Nothing to get.
You're done.
No more work.
Notice how you feel.

—

Practices for Landing
on the Ground

We are learning to allow the ground to carry us.
We are learning to allow our body to be on the earth.
You don't have to hold everything up.
Let the earth hold you.

CONTEMPLATION

Imagine you're looking at a photograph of yourself from a time when you felt grounded—steady, safe, relaxed, at ease. This can be a made-up image or a real memory.

What's the environment like? What surrounds you?

What's under your body? Earth? Flooring?

What do you look like when you feel grounded?

What's your posture?

What does it feel like to be you, when you feel grounded, at home, in your body?

Meditation Experience: Hourglass Meditation

This simple technique uses visualization, breathing, and tension release to help you become more grounded.

- Sit in a comfortable position, eyes open or closed. Take a few long exhales. Notice where your body meets support.
- Bring to mind the image of an hourglass that was just turned upside down, sand emptying from top to bottom.
- Envision your body as an hourglass and drain the "sand" out of your upper body down into your lower body on three exhales:
- Exhale: Let all the heaviness empty from your head, neck, and shoulders. Pause and enjoy your inhale.
- Exhale: Feel the solidity draining from your shoulders and chest down into your belly. Let your inhale expand your torso.
- Exhale: Allow all the sandiness to leave your belly and flow down into your pelvis, legs, and feet. Feel your seat expanding into its outline.
- Let your body *land* on the ground completely.
- Place one hand on your heart and one on your belly. Notice the feeling of your breath under your hands.
- For the next few minutes, allow yourself to stay grounded, as your breath flows in and out of your body.
- You will repeatedly be pulled away from your breath. Each time you drift away, don't make a big deal about it. Simply invite your attention kindly back onto the breath.
- To close, welcome yourself again into your seat, on the ground.

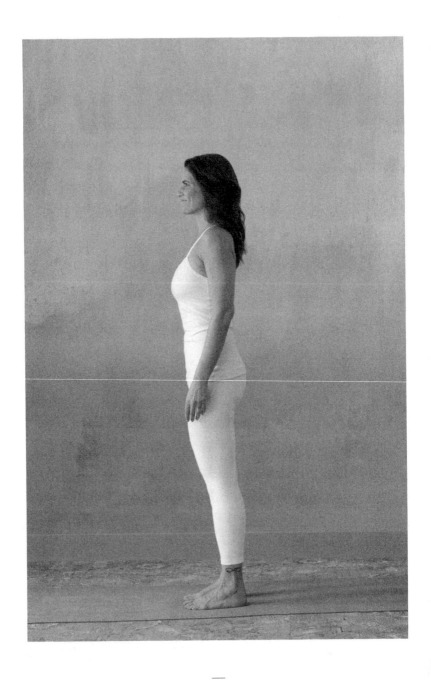

Yoga Experience: Mountain Pose and Mountain Chair Flow

Mountain Pose

- Stand mindfully, feet about hip-distance apart, pelvis stacked over your ankles. Arms by your sides.
- Use 5 to 10 breaths to let all your weight drain down from your top half and into your bottom half.
- Like an hourglass, let the sandy weight in you lower from your head, neck, and shoulders. Drain down from your torso, chest and belly. Feel all your heaviness accumulate in your legs and feet. Like sandbags, let your feet spread beyond their prints. Land completely on the earth.
- As you prepare to close, pause to notice what it feels like to let all your body weight be on the ground.

MOUNTAIN CHAIR FLOW

- Begin in Mountain pose.
- On your inhale, lower your seat into an imaginary chair, as you sweep your arms up to the sky.
- On your exhale, rise back up to Mountain pose while sweeping your arms back down to your sides.
- Enjoy 5 to 10 breaths, flowing between Mountain and Chair.
- To finish, pause in Mountain and enjoy one more full breath.

All the effort in this pose happens in your lower body. Firm the muscles of your seat and back of your thighs; press your feet into the ground. Let your strong lower body carry your light upper body.

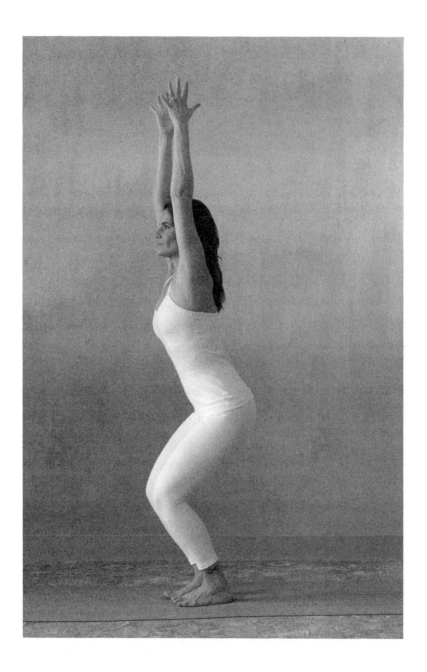

Restorative Yoga Experience: Surfboard

PROPS: Three long rectangle-folded blankets, stacked. One short-rolled blanket.

SET UP

- Place your stack of blankets, vertically, up the center of your mat. You will lie on these like a surfboard.
- Place the rolled blanket across the bottom of your mat to rest the tops of your feet on.
- Begin on all fours over the stacked blankets and lower down onto them—the way you would lie down on a surfboard. A few inches of the top of your thighs comes up onto the blanket stack. Your pelvis, torso, and head are all supported by the blankets. The center of your kneecaps rest on the ground.
- Bring the top of your feet onto your blanket roll.
- Turn your head to one side, with one cheek on your blanket, arms on the ground in the shape of a cactus. If you have any neck issues, try Face Down Variation.

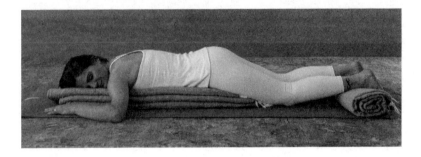

EXPERIENCE SURFBOARD

- Make any adjustments you need to feel more comfort, supported, and relaxed.
- Let your whole body fall into the blankets. Release all the effort in your legs, belly, and arms. No need to hold yourself up. Enjoy a few long breaths to allow your full body weight to drop into your blankets and down into the ground.
- Every few minutes, turn your head to rest on the opposite cheek.
- *Relaxmore* for 5 to 10 minutes.
- To finish, bring your hands under your shoulders, gently firm your belly, and press up onto all fours.
- Slowly come to sitting. Pause and feel your seat on the ground. Welcome your breath into your body.

Face Down Variation: *For those with neck injuries, excessive neck tightness, or carotid artery issues. Fold about 10 inches of the top blanket down, bringing it under your chest and breastbone. Place a support under your forehead, allowing you to arrange your head and neck to sustain a relaxed, natural cervical curve.*

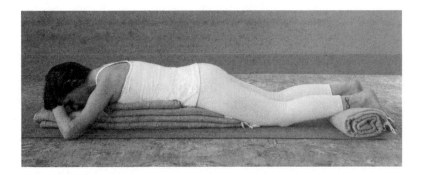

Relaxmore
Land and Relax More

Let your whole body fall into the blankets

No need to hold yourself up.

Exhale, no need to grip your thighs.

Effortless legs.

Exhale, no need to hold on to your belly.

Let your belly rest on your blankets.

The earth will hold you.

Lungs rest on the earth.

Heart free to rest on the earth.

On each exhale, do less.

Allow the earth to hold you up more.

Let your breath flow effortlessly in and out of your body.

Let your breath ripple your spine.

As the ground holds you up, let your breath care for you inside.

Relax more . . . here, now, on the ground.

Welcome your whole self

into this moment.

Journaling Prompts:
Finding Groundedness

What keeps you from feeling grounded?

What helps you feel more grounded?

What can you do to feel more grounded today?

Instant Pause and Reset: Effortless Support

- Come to a relaxed standing position, eyes open, or closed. Use three slow exhales to imagine the sand in you draining down from your head all the way to the earth.
- Exhale: Let your heaviness empty from your head, neck, and shoulders. Welcome your inhale.
- Exhale: Feel the weight drain from your shoulders through your torso all the way to your pelvis. Your inhale to expands you.
- Exhale: Allow all the sand in you to drain down into your legs and feet. Feel your inhale lighten up your whole torso.
- Pause and feel your feet, expanding into their prints. Let your inhale inflate your clear upper body.
- Allow the earth to carry you as you slowly shift your awareness into the space around you.

CHAPTER THREE

Being *Here*

Once we feel welcome in our own lives,
and safe and grounded in our body,
we can start shifting our attention to being here
rather than being there.

THE NIGHT MY SON COULDN'T BREATHE

One spring, my husband and I were sharing a room with then 8-year-old William at one of my favorite mountain resorts. We'd spent the day hiking, and we all turned in early. William had never had a severe reaction to spring pollen, so I wasn't expecting what happened next.

He had been asleep for a few hours when he started to cough—a short dry bark followed by a labored whistling inhale. We tried to settle him, but the cough became worse—quicker and more urgent—like an old man gasping for breath.

We called the hotel paramedics, who showed up with an oxygen mask and brought William to the in-house doctor. We all

—

assumed the oxygen would fix the problem. But it didn't, and I started to panic.

I knew that in order to help my son, I had to calm myself. So I began to consciously focus on my own breathing, which had become as short and shallow as William's.

As my breath slowed and deepened, I immediately started feeling more clear and present. I leaned in toward William, our foreheads touching, and had him breathe with me. William was able to mimic my rhythmic breathing, and after a few minutes he, too, began to relax. Our breath flowed in more easily, and our exhales grew steady and smooth. The panic left his eyes and his cough quieted a bit. We stayed like that, forehead to forehead, until an ambulance came to bring him to the hospital.

When we can't breathe easily, we become anxious, and our mind starts racing out of the present. When a flight attendant tells us to put on our own oxygen mask before we attend to our child, what we're really being told is that we cannot help someone (or ourselves) in an emergency if we are at the mercy of our own anxiety. We become *unable* to thoughtfully attend to what's going on right in front of us.

WE'RE ALL A LITTLE BREATHLESS

The thing about an asthma attack (and breathing in general) is that the *harder* it is to breathe, the *more* anxious we get. Our fear center is alerted, and our body reacts. We become tighter and more rigid, then breathing becomes harder still. This cycle begins and then feeds on itself, leaving us even more tense and anxious.

And when we are in this cycle, it is *neurologically* impossible to feel *okay*.

But this phenomenon does not apply only to asthma. Every time we don't feel *okay*, we are pulled *out* of our relationship with our body and *away* from our breath. And the truth is that most of us are in some version of this cycle all day long.

In fact, we typically don't even realize how minimized our breathing is most of the time. We've gotten so used to feeling restricted, we don't have any idea that it's not the way our body is naturally meant to feel.

Our restricted breath actually begets stress.
It perpetuates the feeling of low-level anxiety
that most of us live with.

The Breath Brings Our Mind Home

Stressful situations will always arise in our life, and sometimes it will feel as if there's no solid ground to support us. Each time we *pause* and replace our attention on our breath, our mind comes "home" to our body. Each time we replace our attention on our breath, we grow more grounded. For a moment, we stop thinking about the future or replaying the past. For a moment, we can stop zipping around trying to make things better.

Paying attention to our breath brings us *here,* into the present, where we are able to notice what's happening within us and around us on a moment-to-moment basis. It's the fastest, most efficient way to draw ourselves out of that cycle of anxiety—out of that cycle of *not-okayness*—and into a state where we feel centered and calm.

HEY, COME BACK HERE!

Thich Nhat Hanh, one of the world's most renowned teachers of mindfulness, tells one of my favorite stories about why it's important to feel ourselves *here*, grounded in the present. Years ago, this Buddhist monk started an "intentional community" in France, a village for people who wanted to focus on living harmoniously with one another and the earth. It has evolved into a retreat community, and every year thousands of people come to practice becoming more present in their lives.

A while back, a television news reporter came to the village to do a story about the community. Before the reporter started his work, Thich Nhat Hanh invited him to join in on their daily walk.

This walk is silent and gentle. Everyone in the community walks together. People are encouraged to pay attention to three things: their feet meeting the earth, the beauty that surrounds them, and the coming and going of their breath.

After that walk, Thich Nhat Hanh asked the reporter how he felt. The reporter said the walk left him exhausted and he had to go take a nap. Thich Nhat Hanh asked how he could be so tired after such an easy, lovely, meandering walk.

But the reporter didn't experience a mindful walk at all. Instead, he had devoted his attention to worrying about his reporting, developing and refining his questions. So at the end of this stroll designed to rejuvenate, he felt spent.

When we're somewhere else rather than *here*, expending our

—

energy on planning for the future or rehashing the past, we feel drained. It's exhausting to be somewhere other than where we are.

Imagine yourself someplace where you are totally at ease—maybe you're on the beach or hiking in the woods; maybe you're in your garden or snuggled in front of a warm fire. Now, imagine being in this place and *really paying attention* to where you are and *how it feels* to be there. We can be in the most relaxing, nourishing place in the world, but if we are busy-minded or fast-forwarding or rewinding to some *other* place, we have a completely different experience.

If we want to develop a sense of well-being, we need to come back *here*. If we want our body to move into the mode of health and healing, we need to come back *here*.

WHY WE DON'T STAY *HERE*

I n addition to our cultural tendency to rewind and fast-forward our days away, another reason we avoid what's right in front of us is that sometimes what's in front of us is not so easy to be with. So we try to make things the way we want them rather than flow with the changes life brings.

We live under the illusion that we can control the events of our lives. Everything we work so tirelessly to construct—from our relationships to our jobs to our identity—can change in an instant. This was made painfully clear when Lisa became ill. For me, her illness was very real proof that we don't ever know for certain what tomorrow will bring.

When we're young, it's easier to embrace change. In fact, unfamiliar experiences are necessary for parts of our brain to develop. But as we get older, we are more naturally drawn to sameness. That is how we're wired. A certain amount of predictability in life helps us feel safe.

The more time I spent with Lisa during the 3 years of her illness, the more tightly I tried to cling to my "ideas" of me. I was a go-getter. I was an athlete. I was a person who needed to keep busy all the time.

I continued to clutch on to *who I was* in an effort to control a world that, to me, felt as if it were spinning out. And while my efforts may have seemed a good idea at the time, I ultimately could not sustain them. Because no matter how much planning or arranging or

—

clinging we do to make ourselves feel secure, there will always be circumstances beyond our control.

This is because the natural order of things is not sameness, but change. We can easily see this in the life cycle of plants and seasons, as buds turn into leaves that then evolve from summer green to autumn gold before they fade and fall to the winter earth. Seasonal changes are something we rely on, even look forward to. Yet we spend a lot of energy trying to resist change in our own life.

But the truth is, *nothing* ever stays the same.

THE BREATH-ANXIETY CONVERSATION

We can become "breathless" in the blink of an eye. In fact, the stress response initiates in about one-twentieth of a second— the time between two heartbeats. So if we feel provoked or humiliated or ashamed, our breath becomes short and shallow instantly, the same way it would if we were frightened and had to sprint from danger. Our shallow breathing signals our fear center that things are *not okay,* and we enter into the cycle of breathlessness begetting anxiety, anxiety begetting bodily tension, and tension begetting breathlessness.

Similarly to the way we can take a physical approach to "feel" grounded, we can also address our anxiety by focusing on what's happening in our body. For example, we know that our psoas muscle tightens when we are stressed. The top of the psoas attaches to our spine right around the diaphragm, and ideally, when we breathe, our spine moves supplely. However, when the psoas contracts into that urgent runner's stance, it pulls on our spine. As a result, the spine moves less fluidly and the area around our diaphragm becomes compressed and constricted. The less freely the spine moves, the less freely the diaphragm moves. The less freely the diaphragm moves, the less easily we breathe.

And the less freely we breathe, the more anxious—and less present—we feel.

The good news: Mindful breathing can break that loop.

When our diaphragm is moving fully and freely, a message is sent through our nervous system that says, "We're safe." In other

—

words, it is our slow, easy breathing that flips the "light switch" in our imaginary "body house." It calms us, letting our brain know that the Survival Room can go offline. And once that switch is flipped, energy can be sourced back to our long-term health and healing rooms. When we slow down our breath and become present, it's like we are recharging ourselves.

Getting grounded and becoming present are practices we do in tandem. We practice feeling our body land on the earth. And then we practice paying attention to the single thing that can unfailingly anchor us in the present moment: our breath.

THE BREATH IS SOMETHING WE ALLOW

Slowing down our breath takes little more than attention. Breathing is not an "activity" we need to accomplish. It is simply a process that we *allow* to happen.

As we practice letting go of effort and feeling the ground support us, we begin to experience the natural rise and fall of the breath. We notice that after an exhale, our lungs spontaneously and organically fill again with air. The breath is simply waiting for more room so that it can fill us. And we can begin to see how our breath is our life partner, always there for us—without question.

Similar to the way we learn to rely on the support of the ground, becoming aware of our partnership with the breath reinforces our experience of connectedness. Of not feeling alone.

Your breath is talking to you all the time. . .

and usually sweetly, if you listen.

Your breath is not the one that's saying,

"Hey, idiot."

Your breath is the one that's saying,

"Hey, I love you."

THE EVER-CONSTANT,
EVER-CHANGING BREATH

There are a few reasons the breath is the perfect tool for becoming present. First, the breath is continual and constant. It gives us the opportunity, over and over, wherever we happen to be, to notice "This is an in breath" and "This is an out breath."

In breath. Out breath.

In. Out.

Second, our breath is never the same. Everyone breathes differently. And every breath is unique. When we observe our breath, in all its variety and nuance, we are practicing sitting quietly with this process that is vital to our life but that is also in a constant state of change.

Every breath is new, and every breath brings us into the present moment.

The breath is our metronome of now.

You don't actually have to make an effort to

breathe. In fact, you have to take away effort.

To inhale, you let the breath come to you.

To exhale, you simply get out of its way.

COME BACK *HERE* AGAIN!

Sometimes I sit in meditation and for the entire time feel really present with my breath. And I think, *"Finally* I'm going to have this same feeling of true presence in just this way every time I sit to meditate." But that's not what happens. Instead, I often find that every 30 seconds or so, like the journalist on Thich Nhat Hahn's walk, I'm thinking about my reporting instead of paying attention to my breath. I've been meditating for 25 years, and this is still true.

The practice isn't to figure out how to *stay* here, it's learning how to come back. Our practice actually begins each and every time we find ourselves *there* instead of *here*. We're learning how to *notice* that we've tripped out and then how to *guide* ourselves back. It doesn't matter how many times we trip out. What matters is that we return.

Here.

Sweetly. Gently. Over and over again.

We're training in returning to our breath in yoga and meditation so that we can return to our breath when we're out in the world. So we can confidently pause and listen to our life with the support of our calming, centering breath.

Listening to Your Breath

Imagine being with someone who loves and supports you—

a friend . . .

a teacher . . .

someone who really means it when they say,

"Sweetheart, you don't have to work so hard.

You can relax. Come relax with me."

Just for right now

there's nothing to get.

Nowhere to go.

It's okay not to work so hard.

Exhale as if all your work is done.

Find the space at the end of your exhale.

Feel that space at the end of your breath.

Even for only one breath.

Allow yourself to feel what it *feels* like

to be done.

Listen to your breath as it comes and goes.

Listen to your inhale as it fills you.

Listen while your breath says to you,

"Hey, come here.

Come be with me.

Let's be together.

Let's be together, here, now."

Practices for Being Here

We are learning to let our breath arrive in our body.
We are learning to be with our breath as it flows.
We are practicing both moving along with
and allowing ourselves to be moved by
our breath as it is actually happening.

CONTEMPLATION

Enjoy a few long deep breaths. Notice what is happening in your immediate space in this moment. Listen. Name a few sounds you hear. What surrounds you? Name a few things you see.

Now shift your attention inward as you continue to be aware of your breath. Ask yourself, "What do I feel like right now? What does my body feel like? My energy level? My mood? My mental state?" Name a few things you notice about yourself in this present moment.

Keeping 50 percent of your attention on your breath and how you feel, expand your awareness back into the space around you.

Notice what it's like to be you, as you are, in this living moment, as it is happening.

Our breath literally moves us, even when we
are at rest. As we inhale, our front spine
naturally unfurls and the chest opens and
expands. As we exhale, the spine naturally
curls in, softly retracting. When we are
relaxed, our spine is rippled by the breath,
the way an underwater sea plant is fluidly
moved by the tide.

MEDITATION EXPERIENCE:
BEING WITH THE FLOW OF YOUR BREATH

This simple technique uses visualization to help you feel more grounded so that you can be present, with your breath, here, now.

- Sit in a comfortable position on the ground or in a chair, eyes open or closed. Pause for a few exhales and notice where your body meets support.

- If you'd like, use the welcoming elevator (pages 18 to 19) or the hourglass (page 39) imagery to help you drain your body weight down into the ground.

- Mentally scan your face and then your body for habitual tension.

- Release any squinting around the eyes, brows, and temples. Let your jaw dangle. No need to grip anywhere in your head, your neck, your shoulders. Everything drains down: down your torso, down through your belly. Let yourself land on the ground completely.

- Now imagine you are sitting on a beach on a calm day, watching the gentle ocean waves rise and fall. Just like the ocean, each wave of our breath fluidly comes and goes, in and out, on its own. We are simply practicing allowing the breath to flow on its own as we witness it. Without expectation, judgment, or changing anything, simply bring your open attention to the coming and going of each breath.

- For more support in staying present with your breath, add a mental mantra—silently chant for the length of your inhale,

---

"*Flowing in*," and for the duration of your exhale, "*Flowing out*." Use these mantras and sit for 5 to 10 minutes *watching* the waves of your breath.

- To close, welcome yourself into your seat. Set an intention to stay with your breath—to stay with yourself—as you transition into your next activity.

Like a raft on a wave, let your mind rest on
the flow of your breath. Stay with your
breath. Your attention will repeatedly drift
away from your breath. That's okay.
Simply *return* to greet your breath,
over and over again.

Yoga Experience: Cat/Cow Flow

Cat/Cow is a flowing yoga exercise. We are practicing synchronizing our movement with the breath. This requires a balance of action and surrender. Move with your breath—and let the breath move you.

- Come to all fours. Your hands slightly wider than your shoulders. Your knees about as wide as your hips.
- Listen for your breath. As your inhale fills you, move into Cow by dropping your belly toward the mat, arching your back. Lift your breastbone forward as you gaze to the horizon or up to the sky.
- As your breath flows out, move with it into Cat. Press down through your hands, gather your belly into your back, and

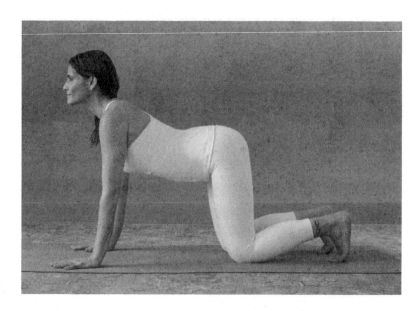

round your spine to the sky. Bring your chin toward your chest as you gaze at your thighs.

- Notice the pause at bottom of your exhale. Enjoy a moment of stillness as you wait for the inhale to flow back into you. Let your breath help move you into Cow.
- Wait for your exhale to help move you back into Cat.
- Continue moving mindfully between Cat and Cow for a minute or two. If you'd like, try this with your eyes closed as you listen inward to your breath.
- Let your spine move like a wave. Liquid, graceful, seamless.
- Like your breath, let your movement be a metronome of now.
- When you are ready to finish, mindfully transition out of the pose.

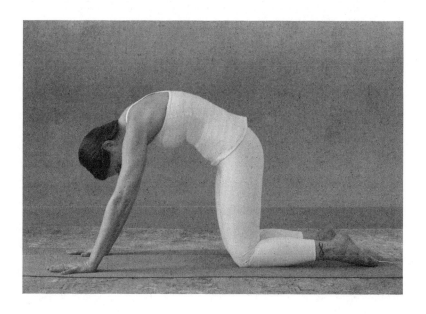

RESTORATIVE YOGA EXPERIENCE:
EASY CHEST OPENER

PROPS: Two long rectangle—folded blankets, stacked. One short-roll blanket. Two blocks. If you'd like, place a blanket over you for warmth.

SET UP

- Prepare support for back. Place the two stacked blankets vertically up the center of your mat, with about a third of the length hanging off the back of your mat.
- Prepare support for leg. Sit on your mat, with your blanket stack behind you. At the front of your mat, place two blocks side by side and lay the short-roll blanket on top of the blocks.
- Bring your legs over the blanket, letting the roll fill in the back of your knee pits. The backs of your heels should rest on your mat.
- Lie down. Hold the corners of your blanket stack to help you stay centered as you slowly lower your back down onto the

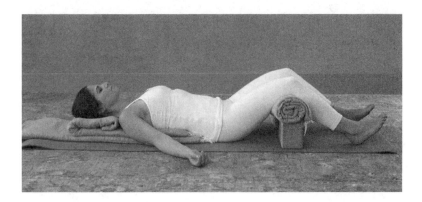

blankets. The blanket stack should fill in the curve of your lower back all the way up to your head. (Your seat is on the mat, not on your blanket.)

- Create head support. Reach back and fold the top blanket under you until it meets your shoulders. Ensure that your neck has a natural cervical curve.
- Bring your arms by your sides, palms down or faceup. Or rest your hands on your belly, elbows on the ground.

EXPERIENCE EASY CHEST OPENER

- Take some time to make any adjustments you need to ensure that you are evenly laid out and comfortable. When you are ready to settle down, enjoy several long breaths to progressively release all of your body weight down toward the ground.
- *Relax more* for 5 to 15 minutes.
- For the last minute of the pose, bring your hands to your belly and feel your palms receive your breath.

  Welcome your caring breath with your caring hands.
  Imagine the breath unraveling any lingering knots inside.

- To close, slowly begin to move in any way that feels good. Then mindfully roll to your side and take your time to press up to a comfortable seated position and pause. Set an intention to stay aware of your breath as you transition out of the pose.

—

Relaxmore
BE HERE AND RELAX MORE

Enjoy a few long breaths
as you slowly scan your mind along the back of your body.
Take your time to notice all the places you feel your body making
contact with support.

Your heels heavy on the ground.
Your legs held up completely.
Your seat dropping into the earth.
Your back spreading across your blankets.
Arms carried by the floor.
Your head resting fully on the ground.

Welcome your breath into your body.
Your breath will soften your belly.
Allow your belly to soften and melt into your back.
Let it pool down into the ground.

Let the space between your ears widen.
The roof of your mouth soften.
Your tongue resting on the floor of your mouth.
Voluminous tongue.
Throat free to fill the neck.

Allow your breath to flow through you.
Feel the rise and fall of your breath moving your torso.

—

Your ribs rippled by your breath.

Collarbones drift on the tide of your breath.

The skin of your chest

floating on the waves of your breath.

Your lungs effortlessly expanding

into the space around them.

Let your mind rest on your breath, in your body.

Welcome your breath with your whole being.

Let yourself flow along with the breath.

Be here with your breath.

JOURNALING PROMPTS: GROWING PRESENT

In what parts of your life—in what situations—do you feel most present?

When you realize you are not present, what do you find yourself doing? Are you doing something habitual like worrying about the future or revisiting a past event? Rushing? Planning? Checking e-mails or social media? Eating?

Fill in the blank: Today, to help myself feel more present more often, I will _____

—

INSTANT PAUSE AND RESET:
BE HERE NOW

Pause and use your breathing to instantly reset your attention and presence several times a day. Keep your eyes open as you turn your attention to your body and breath—to where you are in real time.

- Pause and sense where your body meets the ground. Soften excess squinting and gripping in your face, neck, and shoulders.
- For the next three breaths, silently chant for the length of your inhale, "*I am*," and for the duration of your exhale, "*here now*." Allow the breath to come and go on its own, no effort.
- Pause at the end of your third breath and notice your body meeting support. Notice your breath flowing freely, and open your awareness fully to the immediate space around you. Notice what is in your space—and what is truly happening now.
- Welcome yourself into this moment: Welcome yourself, as you are, *however* you feel, into this moment, as it is.
- Stay with your breath, with yourself, as you move back into your day.

CHAPTER FOUR

How We Hold

We welcome ourselves,

settle onto the ground,

and meet our breath.

Next we pause to notice what's happening

in our body and our mind.

BLOODLETTING

When I was 12 years old, I had mononucleosis and hepatitis, and I had to have blood drawn practically every week for months. I have tiny veins, and it's always been difficult for nurses to access them. They'd wind up using a painful procedure called fishing, which involves poking the needle in and spinning it until it makes contact with the vein. In addition to a lot of black-and-blue marks, I wound up with loads of anxiety about needles that persisted into adulthood.

Several years ago, I had an early-morning appointment to get my annual blood work done. I had to drop William at school and go

—

straight to the lab. Morning is not what I consider our most "grace-ful" time, and on this particular morning, besides our regular strug-gle of getting up and out the door, William and I had gotten into an argument. When I arrived at the lab, I was cranky and stressed.

The nurse started looking for my vein and, as usual, I tried to take charge. "Can you *please* use the butterfly needle and can you use *this* vein?" I asked, pointing to a spot that had worked in the past.

She inserted the needle where I'd instructed. Nothing hap-pened. She was in the vein, but no blood was coming out. I felt myself getting even more stressed than I already was, worrying that this blood draw was going to end up like every other one—prolonged and painful.

I expected the nurse to start fishing, but she didn't. Unlike the nurses of my childhood, she did not seem to be worried about how much time this might take. She just sat with me, looking into my eyes with a serene, benevolent smile. "Honey, relax," she said to me (the yoga teacher!). "Take a deep breath."

Her sweetness calmed me. I took a few breaths and ultimately filled three vials.

INTRODUCING TENSION

Normally, when a needle enters a vein, blood flows immediately. But when we are stressed, our muscles contract and many of our systems are compromised. I was so bound up emotionally that morning, the tension in my body affected my blood flow.

In my experience, muscle *tension* is different from muscle tightness. Tightness is when you use a muscle in some way and it doesn't return to its resting length, say from exercising or gardening or moving heavy furniture. *Tension* usually contains a psychological or emotional component. For example, if I'm driving on an icy highway and I need to stay alert to possible danger, I turn down the radio and sit more rigidly in my seat. After a while, my shoulders ache. That's tension. We're armoring up because we feel vulnerable in some way.

Once we're out of the car, our shoulders usually release. Muscle tightness responds to stretching; muscle tension responds to feeling safe.

Tension can be long-standing and result from something physical, like the way we try to protect ourselves from a past injury. Or it might accumulate as a result of an old hurt—the way we may slouch because we were made fun of in third grade. Maybe it's something we carry from living in a house where parents were always fighting or from living in a country that's in constant strife.

Hunched shoulders, fisted hands, protruding chests, jutting chins, and even collapsed posture can be indicators that somewhere in our past we felt threatened and built layers of muscular tension as a defense.

But tension can also arise from something new, like getting into a fight with someone we love or caring for someone who is ill. Our body is responding to feeling provoked or overwhelmed, to feeling left out or unloved. Tension is the way we store what we don't want to feel, and it's also the way we shield ourselves from what we don't want to take in.

—

We feel threatened, so we harden.

Whether we're carrying emotions from our past or emotions from this morning, whether we're feeling pushed into the future or pulled into the past, whether we're reacting to dangerous road conditions or receiving tough news from a doctor, if our nervous system is triggered regularly and our stress hormones don't have the chance to dissipate quickly enough to return to a calm state, we can end up with tension.

We all harden ourselves,

every single day.

We may not know it as it's happening,

but we will undoubtedly experience its

effects.

Tension is the stress response

finding a home in our body.

THE TENSION STORY

Living with tension is like getting dressed to go to a party in clothes that are two sizes too small. Everything feels constricted. It's *uncomfortable*. I don't know about you, but if I'm wearing something even *one* size too small, I feel annoyed and grumpy. It's hard to enjoy what I'm doing. I'm at this party with all the people I really want to spend time with, and I can't pay attention to them. In fact, I can't pay attention to much of anything except my own discomfort.

Yet these "too-tight clothes" are what we're wearing every day. We live in them. In fact, most of us even sleep in them.

This is not an exaggeration. Before I learned how to relax deeply, I could go a whole night without ever giving my full weight to my mattress. I'd be lying down, but at the same time I was *holding* myself off the bed. I even started noticing this same *holding* when I brushed my teeth or blow-dried my hair. It was a revelation to learn that I could get myself ready every day without my shoulders needing to be up near my ears.

Throughout the day, we hold ourselves in a constant state of alertness, as if we don't believe that whatever is underneath us is truly supporting us. We do not feel at ease in our body, and we compensate for that in ways that are so automatic they've become our "normal."

The way we hold ourselves,

and the armor we engage

keep us separate, hard,

and unable to release into the support

available to us.

—

Living in Too-Tight Clothes

It's probably no surprise that this constricted state we're often in does not serve our well-being.

When our "inner clothes" are too tight, everything inside us remains bound up. Most of the time, our tension reveals itself through long-term muscle pain—backaches, tightness in our shoulders, stiffness in our hips. But it's also at the root of why many of us simply don't feel *good*. Our organs are restricted. The systems in our body don't work as well. This is what happened during my blood test. The needle was in my vein, yet the blood did not move. However, as the nurse's kind demeanor made me feel safe and cared for, I could let myself breathe and relax.

My breath flipped the switch out of the stress response. I stopped worrying about whether the nurse was going to hurt me, and I arrived into the present moment to meet her sweet smile. I stopped rewinding back to my fight with my son and fast-forwarding to how black and blue this was likely to leave me. My body released its holding, and some tension fell away.

No fishing. No pushing or prodding. The only thing she did was help set the conditions that allowed me to release the way I was holding myself.

But sometimes it's not so easy to just relax into our "now."

Imagine what it would be like wearing those too-tight clothes and, instead of being at a party, you were somewhere you didn't want to be at all. Imagine trying to endure a difficult encounter in your too-tight clothes when there's not one single thing around you that helps you feel okay. I will freely admit that when I'm in a situation like that, my mind starts zipping to a whole host of other places that either distract me or feed my misery.

We all have a tendency to pay lots of attention to the thoughts that arise as soon as things don't feel okay. And believe me, this does nothing to loosen our too-tight clothes. So we need to practice attending to our thoughts in a slightly different way—a habit that's easier to develop once we understand the nature of how our mind works.

Our Brain Is a Thought Factory

The first thing we need to realize is how *much* we think. We are a thinking species, and our brain is built to generate thought constantly—meaning nonstop. By some estimates, we have more than 50,000 thoughts per day. When we pay attention to our thought stream, we become aware that we tend to start little conversations with our many thoughts. Plenty of our thoughts are "easy" and don't carry much weight—*I have to take out the garbage . . . It's cold in here . . . What should I have for lunch?* But other thoughts trigger memories or feelings that draw us into deeper conversations.

We take our original thought and start *adding on* to it. And in doing so, *we* begin to give the whole thought stream more weight. Getting tangled up in thoughts like this is so natural, we are barely aware it's happening.

Here's an example of my conversation with my thoughts at the blood lab:

ME: No blood is coming out.

ME: Why isn't that spot working? That spot always works . . .

ME: Ugh, is she going to start poking me?

ME: I hate getting my blood drawn.

ME: She's not going to find the right spot.

ME: Why won't it flow?

ME: Please just let this be over.

Often our original thought is neutral before we start the dialogue. "No blood is coming out" is simply an objective description of what was happening in that one moment. But we hook into that thought and pile on lots of other things—things that once happened or might happen—and before we know it, a compelling conversation is taking place in our head.

We all have our own little dialogues that we easily slip into. Once we become aware of our tendency to start these conversations, we can see how automatically they begin and how "normal" they feel. It doesn't matter what form our particular conversation might take— dialoguing with our thoughts like this usually means we're zipping away from *here*. And that rarely makes anything *truly* better.

HITTING REPLAY

According to current research, on average more than 90 percent of our daily thoughts tend to be *repeats*. Meaning we spend almost all of our time thinking thoughts we've had before. Maybe we're replaying a recent argument, rehashing every possible thing we could have said. Or maybe we keep revisiting some fantasy that distracts us from our dreary job. Our repeat thoughts are one of the main ways we zip away from *here,* usually without even noticing.

What makes this especially troubling is that studies show upwards of 80 percent of our repeat thoughts tend to be *negative* in nature.

These thoughts are usually ones that remind us how we need to *be better* and *do more.* That remind us how we feel inadequate or ashamed, powerless or hurt. The thoughts we return to are *not* the ones that make us feel spacious, worthy, and alive. They're the ones our mind considers threatening.

This tendency is not because we're defective or gloomy. It, too, is a function of our evolutionary design to keep ourselves safe.

When we're primed to protect ourselves, our mind tends to look for whatever else might be dangerous—whatever else might leave us feeling *not okay.* Our thought generator is preprogramed to start offering lots of possibilities: "Uh-oh, what if *some other bad thing* happens?" and "Hey, don't forget about *this* awful possibility!" Because it would be unwise to let our guard down before the coast is clear.

When our thoughts carry some emotional weight and trigger feelings, we start conversations with them. We *add on.* We keep the dialogue going, end up making the thoughts weightier still, and add to our tension without even realizing it.

But it doesn't need to be like this.

—

THE 90-SECOND RULE

Neuroscientist and brain researcher Jill Bolte Taylor describes a phenomenon she came to understand after she'd suffered a stroke and was working to recover her own brain function. She was studying what happens physiologically when we "think" and discovered that our triggering, weighty thoughts have a natural life span of only about 90 seconds—as long as we do not engage with them. In other words, if we have a potentially stressful thought—"No blood is coming out"—and we simply observe that thought without "adding on," the feelings that are stirred up will typically rise, crest, and dissipate naturally in about a minute and a half.

Ninety seconds can feel like a long time if we're stirred up emotionally. But the beauty of this knowledge is that we can begin to see for ourselves that our feelings often pass quickly if we don't feed them with attention.

Because I was used to being hurt and scared in the blood lab, I automatically got sucked into an internal conversation I'd had dozens of times before.

Most conversations usually start just like this, when something from the past gets triggered. But not always. Conversations can also be triggered by present-moment circumstances, when we feel embarrassed, insulted, or ashamed, or when things are not going as we expected. Sometimes we hook into some distracting thought that simply seems interesting or titillating or somehow holds the promise of being better than *here*.

Whether our thoughts are good or bad or something in between, when we engage them in conversation, unconsciously or on purpose, we're making them more solid. Whether we intend to or not, we're inviting them to stay.

When we notice the pattern of our thoughts,

we can see how they seem so solid at first

but how their nature is to dissolve into

another thought,

and then another,

and then another.

PAUSING TO NOTICE

R ather than having a conversation with our thoughts, we are going to practice just noticing them. Because understanding how our mind works sets the groundwork for noticing where tension resides in our body.

Noticing is softer and quieter than looking. It's not something we *do* as much as something we allow ourselves to *receive*. Noticing is that unassuming, nonjudgmental place in which we're not yet responding. We're simply giving gentle attention to what's happening. This is an important distinction because, remember, those conversations we start automatically come from the place where we react out of habit—and our habitual reactions tend to create even more tension.

But as gentle as noticing is, it is still a skill—something that comes more easily with practice.

We begin with *noticing* what is going on in our mind, because once we're aware of the conversations we tend to start, we can see how effortlessly they come about. But ultimately we work with the mind and body together because our conversations can start in either place, with thoughts and feelings or with physical sensations. Noticing allows us to meet our bodily tension without judgment, without instantly adding on.

Instead of "Oh, no! No blood is coming out!" we can say to ourselves, "Oh, look at that. There's no blood."

NOTICING WHERE WE HOLD

To loosen our "too-tight clothing," we need to release the places we hold tension. But before we can release *how* we hold, we have to discover *where* we hold. This can be tricky at first; it isn't always obvious where our tension resides. We're so used to living with it, we can *think* we are relaxed while, in fact, we are still harboring tension.

Just noticing where our tension is hiding in our body sets the conditions for change.

When I was a kid, I would go to get my teeth cleaned and the hygienist would give me a packet of little red Colgate tablets to take home. I'd brush, chew on a tablet, rinse, and spit, and any place that the dark red pigment adhered to my teeth was where I'd missed brushing—that was where the plaque remained. Once I began to see the plaque, I could go back to those areas with more attention.

Our tension is a little like plaque, starting off as a kind of shield and ultimately adhering to the places we've stored difficult feelings in our body. It gets stronger and tougher as time goes on. And, like plaque, sometimes it's not so easy to see.

We discover where our tension lives by using our relaxation practice specifically to *notice* not only where we're holding ourselves "off the mattress" but also to notice what conversations emerge along *with* our discovery.

We allow ourselves to feel welcome, grounded, and present, and we relax our body so we can *notice* all the spots where, despite the support underneath us, we're still holding. That's where our tension lives.

Gently noticing the ways that we hold ourselves, without thinking we have to make it better or make it different, is actually a way we can care for ourselves. It sends our mind a signal that right now, in this moment, we're okay.

And once we start feeling safe enough to simply *notice* what arises within us, we are setting the conditions to replace our autopilot conversations with responses that support our well-being.

How We Hold

Let your body land on the ground.
Let your breath arrive in your body.
Let your mind rest in your body.
Notice.

Slowly, kindly, scan your body with your mind.
On each inhale, slide your awareness into a single area and
offer your caring attention.
And on each exhale, pause to listen openly.
Notice anything this area holds.
No judgment. Just listen.

Scan slowly, sweetly, starting at your head.
Inhaling, slide your awareness into your eyes.
Exhaling, relax your attention on your eyes.
Inhaling, notice your temples.
Exhaling, listen openly to your temples.
Continue with your ears, cheeks, jaw.
Your lips, tongue, and throat.
Your whole head and neck.
Your upper back, shoulders, arms, and hands.
Your collarbones and breastbone,
solar plexus and middle back.
The outline of your entire rib cage.
The inner lining of your entire rib cage.

—

Your lungs, heart, and belly.

Your whole upper body.

Inside your pelvis.

Your thighs, lower legs, and feet

Your whole lower body.

The outline of your whole body

The inner volume of your whole body.

Notice the *whole* of you.

On your inhale, offer your whole self gentle attention.

On your exhale, listen openly to your whole self.

Practices for Noticing How
We Hold

We are practicing noticing our thoughts, feelings, and sensations
and relaxing with them rather than adding on.
We are learning to notice when, how, and where we tense up,
and rather than judging what we find, we are practicing relaxing with it.

CONTEMPLATION

Imagine you're at a special gathering with some of your dearest people in an environment you love. Notice the details: Where are you? Who is there with you? Now, imagine interacting with your dear company. What would your body feel like? Your breath? Your mind?

Now reimagine yourself at this same event, but you're wearing clothing two sizes too small. What would it feel like to be you in your tight clothing at this gathering? How would your body feel? Your breath? Your mind? What kind of inner dialogue would you be having? How would you act toward your dear ones?

Pause for a few deep breaths and imagine you could go put on your *most comfortable* clothing and reenter the gathering. How would this shift your experience?

MEDITATION EXPERIENCE:
NOTICING AND LABELING

Labeling allows you to acknowledge your feelings and thoughts without having to continue the conversation.

- Sit in a comfortable position, Close your eyes, if you wish. Pause for a few exhales and notice where your body meets support.
- If you'd like, use the hourglass (page 39) imagery to help you drain your body weight down into the ground.
- Observe the flow of your breath. Rest your gentle attention on each breath as it comes and goes on its own.
- Once you notice that you are caught in *thinking*, simply *label* the content or quality of your thought: *planning, worrying, remembering, fixing, fantasizing, sleepy, bored, sad, angry, disappointed, titillated, joyful*, or just plain *"thinking."*
- It doesn't matter how long you've been "away" or what you've been thinking—caringly label it, and then kindly point your attention back to your breath. The practice is learning to come back.
- Sit for 5 to 20 minutes simply observing your breath, noticing and labeling your thoughts, and returning to your breath over and over again.
- To close, pause and set an intention to stay with yourself as you move out of the meditation.

—

Remember, the practice is not to stop your thinking. The practice is to notice when you are no longer with your breath and instead are in a conversation with your thoughts. There is no good or bad here. You are simply giving yourself permission to notice the conversation. You don't have to figure anything out or even finish the conversation right now. You also don't need to forcibly shut the conversation down. Remind yourself that, like your breath, your thoughts and emotions will rise and fall. The energy of a thought will crest and dissipate, like a wave. If you notice it rather than hold on to it in some way, it will loosen its grip on you.

YOGA EXPERIENCE: TREE

B alancing in Tree pose is not about holding things still. Trees sway naturally. However, if you need extra support, do this near a wall or rest your hand on the back of a chair.

- Settle into Mountain pose, allowing your body to land on the earth completely.
- Bring your hands to the rim of your pelvis.
- To help keep your balance, rest your eyes softly on a still point 4 or 5 feet in front of you.
- Shift your weight to your left leg and foot.
- Bring your right heel up onto your left ankle, the ball of your right foot remaining on to the floor.
- Center your pelvis directly over your left foot. Ensure that your hips are the same height.
- If you feel stable, bring the entire sole of your right foot onto your calf or up onto your inner thigh. Press your right foot and left leg equally against each other.
- If you'd like, bring your hands to prayer at your chest or reach your prayer to the sky.
- Like a tree, root down, lengthening from your leg down into your foot down into the ground. Allow your ribs to be moved by your breath, the way branches move with the wind. Trust your strong standing leg to support you.
- For up to 10 breaths, practice noticing what happens in your body, mind, and breath when you feel unsteady. What tightens?

—

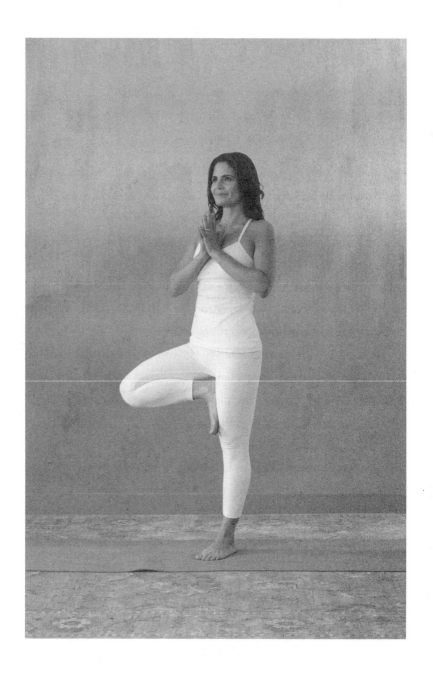

What is your inner dialogue? How do you "hold on"? Simply notice, without judgment, what you are "adding on" to this situation and kindly bring yourself back to your breath.

- To release the pose, step back into Mountain. Repeat on the opposite side.

In Tree pose we are not making a statue of a tree or mimicking a petrified tree. Rather, we are learning to notice how we "hold on," how we overeffort to keep control when we feel wobbly.

When things feel shaky, we shift into survival mode. Our breath grows shallow; our body tenses. When we try to hold things in place, we stiffen. And when we are rigid, there is more potential to get hurt if we fall. When we can notice how we hold on—how we separate—we can then learn to pause, reconnect with the ground and allow the breath to flow more freely. This will help us relax with our sways and wobbles rather than resist them.

—

Restorative Yoga Experience:
Legs up on a Chair

This restorative pose is known to calm and quiet the mind and promote a feeling of groundedness in the body. It is also helpful in relieving excess tension in the back and psoas.

PROPS: A chair, couch, or ottoman. Two small towels for head and neck support. And if you wish, a blanket for warmth or for extra comfort under the body.

SET UP

- Sit with your left hip facing the front of your chair.
- Slowly lower down onto your right side, keeping your knees bent.

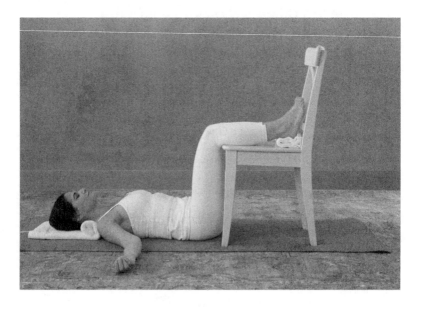

- Mindfully roll onto your back as you bring your legs up on the chair. Rest your legs on the chair's seat, making sure they are supported from the backs of the knees to the heels.
- If you need head support, place a rolled towel under your neck and a folded towel under your head.
- Rest your arms by your sides, either palms down (calming) or palms up (expanding). You may prefer to rest your hands on your belly, elbows on the floor.
- Make any adjustments you need to ensure you are evenly laid out and comfortable.

SETTLE IN

- Take several long breaths, as you progressively release all of your body weight down onto the ground.
- *Relaxmore* for 5 to 15 minutes.
- For the last few breaths, bring your hands to your belly and feel your palms receive your breath. Imagine the breath loosening any lingering hardness inside.
- To come out of the pose, bring your knees in toward your belly and roll to your side, making a pillow with the arm under your head. Relax onto your side completely for a minute.
- Take your time to come to a comfortable seat and close your practice.

—

Relaxmore
Notice and Relax More

Let your body land.
Let your breath arrive in your body.
Let your mind rest in your body.
Notice.

Slowly, kindly, scan your body with your mind,
offering your caring attention.
Gently listen inward to each body part.
Notice where your body holds, where you hold on.
Welcome a deep breath and relax more,

Release a few long exhales through your mouth.

Let your legs relax completely.
Thigh muscles do not need to work.
Effortless thighs.

Let your pelvis drop into the earth.
Earth cradling your pelvis.

Let your belly fall into your back.
Effortless belly.

Allow your back to spread across the floor.
Feel the ground meeting your back.

Welcome your breath into your body.
Let the breath soften your belly more.
Let your breath soften your shoulders more.

—

Let your heart rest into your back.

Let your head rest heavily on the earth.
The ground will hold your head completely.

Temples soften.
Eyes fall into their sockets.
Space between your ears *infinite*.
Tongue voluminous, jaw unhinged.

Your whole body dropping into the earth.
The earth welcomes your weight.
Welcome your breath in your body.
Over and over again.

JOURNALING PROMPTS:
MEETING YOUR TENSION

Recall a time when you felt particularly tense and write about it with as much detail as possible: Where are you? Are you engaged in any particular activity? Are you with anyone?

When you are stressed, is there an area of your body that habitually holds tension—shoulders, jaw, chest, belly? Where does tension live in your body?

Pick one area of tension in your body. If this area of tension could talk, what would it say to you? Write a letter from your tension to you.

Next, can you caringly let your tension know that you've noticed it and that you are paying attention to it? Write a thank-you note to your tension for "protecting" you. Let it know that you'd like to make room for more breath, ease, and healing into your body, mind, and life.

Instant Pause and Reset: Label and Let It Be

Pause to instantly reset your attention several times a day. Take a moment to *notice* the activity in your mind and body. Notice if you are "somewhere else," doing "something else." And draw yourself back into the present.

- Pause and sense where your body meets the ground. Soften excess squinting and gripping in your face, neck, and shoulders. Let yourself land completely.
- *Notice* what is going on in your mind and body right now. Label whatever you find . . . are you planning, worrying, sleepy, sad, happy. Maybe your body is achy, tight, or energized. It doesn't matter what you find, you are just taking a moment to notice how you are and to *label it and let it be.*
- Kindly bring your attention to your next three breaths and mentally chant for the length of your inhale, "*I am*" and for the duration of your exhale, "*here now.*" *I am, here now.*
- Pause at the end of your third breath and notice your body and how you are meeting support. Open your awareness fully to the immediate space around you.
- Welcome yourself into the moment just as you are. Slowly continue into your next activity.

CHAPTER FIVE

Making Space

Like our noticing,
like our trust in the support of the ground,
like our breath,
releasing tension is not something we do.
It's something we allow.

MY FIRST TEARY SAVASANA

After I'd run a marathon, after I'd been ill from chronic fatigue, after I'd been pushing myself at my job and pep-talking myself through life, my boyfriend and I were on the verge of breaking up. And I felt absolutely depleted.

Walking home from work one night, I saw the small bronze sign of a nearby yoga studio—a sign I'd passed hundreds of times before. Without any real plan, I turned into the doorway. Although I'd taken a yoga class or two in college, and occasionally with my mother at her health club when I was a child, I'd never been to an actual yoga studio before. It was 1993, and there were maybe five such studios in all of Manhattan. I rode the small elevator up to the fourth floor and had my very first transformational yoga experience. As an athlete, I was able to move through the 2 hours' worth of poses. But at the end, during Savasana (the final relaxation), I lay on my blue foamy mat and unexpectedly began to sob.

I knew I was tight from years of sports, but it wasn't until that moment that I realized that under the tightness I'd lived with from pushing myself around—muscling through everything I encountered without ever taking a rest—was also a deep and pervasive tension that came from the way I held myself together.

Tension is who you think you should be.

Relaxation is who you are.

—Chinese proverb

THE ART OF RELAXATION

Most of us believe that the way to relax is to step away from our lives. To drop down on the couch and zone out. However, plopping on the couch doesn't address the long-held tension in our body—tension that creates the pain and disease we chase after with therapies and medication.

Releasing tension is the act of consciously making space for *whatever it is we're holding*.

Making space is not complicated, but it's not something most of us are used to. In fact, we're used to doing the opposite, contracting and protecting. So, making space is a skill we must practice.

There are a few essential components to releasing tension:

- We need to feel safe and grounded.
- We need to be present enough to notice where our tension is.
- We need to *allow* what arises and *not add on*.
- And we need to do all of this in such a gentle, kind, friendly way that our body and mind feel like it's all okay.

Releasing tension starts like this: "Hmm, there's that tightness in my right shoulder. Look at that, here it is again." Whatever shows up, we simply notice it, then send it a little more space with our breath.

SPACE = BIGGER, SOFTER

When I was kid, my friends and I used to lie down on the driveway and draw chalk outlines around each other's bodies. It was fun to stand up and see what kind of space our body took up on the ground.

Imagine lying inside your own outline, and, with an exhale, you release all the ways you're holding yourself. You let go of how you're holding yourself up. You let go of how you're holding yourself together. You *allow* yourself to be held by the ground. Imagine how your physical body might spread out. Imagine how your shape might expand beyond your outline. You'd feel bigger. Softer. More spacious.

Making space means allowing everything a little more room. To experience our own spaciousness, we don't have be better and do more. We have to *be here* and *do less*.

MEETING OUR STILLNESS

I remember laying down on my mat during that first teary Savasana, thinking I was being exactly the person I was supposed to be—a strong young woman setting goals and achieving them, getting things done. Of course I did: this is how most of us are trained by practically every one of our role models. But when my motorboat finally stopped zipping and I encountered my stillness, it didn't feel very good. Because when my busy mind quieted down—really quieted down—I realized that the tension I was holding in my body came not only from how much I was racing all the time but also from old feelings I'd tucked away.

When I was growing up, my father was not an easy person to be around. He was the guy who'd drive 100 miles per hour on Main Street, cutting people off. He was the guy who scammed the parking spot someone was waiting patiently for. Dad would walk into the house after work holding a gum wrapper he'd found on our driveway, and my brothers and I would brace ourselves for his fury—and our punishment.

My father controlled everything in our house, from the thermostat to the emotional climate. I learned early on how important it was to yield to him. Because when he felt out of control of *his* world, I did not feel safe. Still, I yearned for his love.

As a young girl, I remember writing in my diary: "Why does he treat me this way? I deserve better than this. How can *I* be better so he will love me?"

CONVERSATIONS WITH MY FATHER

The conversations I had in my mind about my father took up a lot of my thinking time. This dialogue felt urgent and true, but more important, it became "me." My "story" developed—the one where I must not be good enough, and to get my father to pay me the kind of loving attention I wanted, I had to be *better*. I pushed myself daily—in sports, in school, at my job. I spent all my time achieving, and these achievements became who I was in the world.

Perhaps my biggest achievement in my mind was my ability to endure my father's tyranny, and I wore that like a badge of honor. It made me feel strong, and that, too, became who I was.

We're often not consciously aware of these old foundational conversations that live inside us—how they define us, and how they often control us. I certainly wasn't.

But during that first Savasana, as I began to release some of how I was holding myself, I started feeling things I'd been protecting myself from for years. Old hurts bubbled up from under my tense muscles, and it gave me my first glimpse into how exhausting it was to hold myself together.

Making Space versus "Letting Go"

Creating space is different from "letting things go."

I once believed I needed to let go of certain things, because I thought the stuff I was holding on to must be "bad" parts of me. That perspective reinforced the idea that I had to get rid of something or I wouldn't be *okay*. It felt like a little war was going on inside me.

I am no longer fond of the concept of letting things go because it implies that we need to eliminate something from our life, and that idea can create *more* tension. The truth is, we are all a walking summary of our life experiences—everything we've taken in, good and bad.

So instead of trying to "let things go," I invite my students to "let things be." This is the attitude from which we can make space. Rather than pushing parts of us away, we are instead creating an environment that allows us to simply loosen our grip. We don't have to fix anything. All we're doing is bringing tender, nonjudgmental attention to our body and making room for *whatever* is living there. This is how the process of sustainable change begins.

Nothing ever goes away

until it teaches us

what we need to know.

--Pema Chödrön

Our Salty Solution

Imagine pouring a tablespoon of salt into a shot glass filled with water. If you drank what was in that glass, it would taste very, very salty.

Now imagine taking that same tablespoon of salt and pouring it into a big mug full of water. Still salty, but not nearly as salty as the shot glass.

Same salt into a bucket? The solution is less salty. Into a bathtub? Less salty still.

Our challenging thoughts, feelings, and experiences—that's our "salt." My "story" about my difficult relationship with my father is my salt. There's no way I can go back and change what happened in my past; it is always with me. So I'm just trying to make space for it.

The tension we hold in our body keeps our salt container small.

Imagine that single tablespoon of salt poured into a lake. *It's the same amount of salt*, but it has nowhere near the concentration as the shot glass or even the bathtub. In a shot glass, that salty water is undrinkable. But in a bathtub it is barely noticeable. It can even soften the water.

The more diluted our salt is, the less it triggers us. The less it stings. When we have more space for our salt to dissolve, it's easier to make wise, compassionate choices for ourselves.

The truth is, we all have a vastness within us that can contain all our salt. But we often don't experience it because when we loosen our grip, we get scared and tighten up again.

So we practice. We actively make room in our body for all the things we happen to come across. We might notice a pain in our hip, and we practice noticing that feeling with kindness rather than judgment. We might feel agitated or bored or irritable or sad, and we practice paying attention to our breath as these things come up, rather than adding on. We attend to our feelings the way we attend to our breath, allowing them to rise and fall without making them into a story. *Adding on* makes the space more crowded. So we practice just letting things *be*.

That sounds like it should be simple, right? But unfortunately, when we begin to actually relax, things can sometimes get in our way.

WE FEEL OUT OF CONTROL

Years ago, I worked privately with a client who was the CEO of a big, international company. He was a powerful man, responsible for a lot of people as well as the successes and failures of his business. Even after an accident that left him paralyzed and in a wheelchair, he did not slow down in his demanding job. He thrived on being in control, and then, after the accident, he *needed* to be in control. Still, his wife worried about his stress and called me to work with him.

I took him through a relaxation practice that allowed him to release some of his deeply held tension, and initially, he said it was divine. At the end of our first session, he told me he felt relief for the first time in years.

But after a few classes, the very *idea* of relaxing began to cause him anxiety. For him, letting his guard down made him feel as if he would lose his power in the world. He loved *being* relaxed, but at the same time, he hated the process of relaxing. This is not unusual. Being at ease can be alarming if we're used to being "in control." And initially, it may not feel so good.

WE FEEL OUR VULNERABILITY

The "plaque" we're attending to when we begin to relax is there to protect something. Something we either weren't ready to deal with or couldn't deal with. Maybe it was a physical trauma. Maybe it was not enough food on the plate. Maybe it was getting yelled at by the boss. It could be anything that was a big deal to us. In fact, whatever we are protecting might not be a big deal to anybody else—that doesn't matter. If it's a big deal to us, it gets a nice little safe spot.

When we release our tension, what had been protected becomes exposed. Usually, we've done such a good job shielding ourselves that it leaves us feeling very vulnerable when we shed some armor. And when we sense our vulnerability, we feel the need to protect ourselves even more.

Here again, the very act of softening may create the impulse to shield ourselves anew.

Feeling vulnerable makes us tense.

But also the more we try to avoid feeling

vulnerability, the more tense we get.

WE START TO CLING

B esides our aversion to feeling out of control or feeling vulnerable, it can be scary to discover that much of our tension is made up of conversations that we've been having in our mind for years—our stories about what might happen or what should have happened or what we're afraid won't ever happen. And even though these stories may cause us pain, we cling to them.

There's a Buddhist fable I love about how we cling.

A monk is walking down a path and hears wailing in the distance. The monk follows the sound and finds a man hugging a thorn bush, screaming from the pain. The man and the bush appear to be entwined, so the monk tries to help. He tells the man that if he works very slowly and carefully, one body part at a time, he can free himself.

The man gently and methodically disengages himself from the bush that's causing all his suffering, and he moans with happiness.

"I'm free! I feel great! Thank you!" he says to the monk.

Then suddenly, the man becomes uneasy. His eyes narrow in suspicion. "Wait a minute!" he says, spinning toward the monk. "You can't have this bush! It's mine!"

And he wraps himself around it anew.

It feels good to alleviate our suffering. And it also doesn't feel good. Because the "salt" that causes our suffering is familiar. It's *ours*. And we are built to be most comfortable around what's familiar. We might sometimes think we're crazy when we cling to ideas, feelings, and behavior that we know make us feel bad. But it's not crazy. It's the natural habit we've developed as a means of protecting ourselves. We're wired to want to feel in control.

A Better Solution

Creating space does not mean increasing the distance between you and whatever makes you uneasy. While that may seem like a good idea, it's only a short-term solution.

Rather, we create space by training ourselves to recognize a triggering moment and then choose to relax on purpose.

However, most of us can't simply "relax" on command. Instead, we need to work gently with the *design* of our nervous system.

It's like an airplane that's about to land. Before it can touch down, it needs to receive a message: "Welcome! It's safe to land here."

So even if it's just a little moment of welcoming—welcoming our breath into our body—we're setting the conditions to feel that it's okay to *come down* here.

Once we feel supported by the ground, we can gently allow in more breath. Our easy breath reinforces to our nervous system that we're safe, and our mind can begin to shift into a new conversation: "I'm okay here on the ground—with *whatever* my conditions are."

WHY MAKE SPACE?

Initially, releasing tension was nerve-racking for me. Who will I be if I let down my guard and see what's under all my armor? If I don't cling to my "strength," what will be left of me?

You may rightly ask: Why practice yoga on this level? Why not simply master some headstands and be done with it?

Because, for most of us, it's debilitating to live in a body that's holding tension. It's draining to live a life in which we're constantly responding to emotional triggers in ways that sabotage our health and well-being.

It's far more exhausting to live in armor than it is to discover how to truly relax. When we start to release tension, we see results almost immediately. The time we spend in the relaxation response provides the resources that make relaxing in the face of an emotional challenge much easier.

Initially it might feel scary, but eventually you'll find yourself in front of an old trigger and the salt won't sting so much.

And then one day, you may not feel the salt at all.

Making Space

Take a moment to gather yourself here.
Let your body land on the ground.
Let your breath arrive in your body.
Let your mind rest on your breath in your body.
Here, now.

Welcome the breath with a receptive belly.
Your breath will gently unravel the tension it meets.
Your breath will tenderly expand you inside.
Allow your breath to unwind you,
unfurl you.

Let yourself be opened by your breath.
Allow your breath to rise and fall.
Let it flow in and out of you,
on its own,
softening everything in its path.
Expanding you.

You're bigger than you think you are.

—

Practices for Making Space

We are learning to soften and make space
for everything to rise and fall.
We are practicing allowing ourselves to expand.

CONTEMPLATION

Close your eyes. Imagine a photograph of a wide-open sky. Perhaps this sky opens over the infinite ocean or rises above a vast green field. This could be a place you have visited before, a photo you have seen in a magazine, or an image you're creating in your mind.

Imagine transporting yourself to this place, gazing out at the endless sky.

Notice as many details as possible. Where are you? What is the quality of light? What is underneath your body? What sounds or scents would be there? What would it feel like in your body while you're looking out into this openness? What would it feel like in your mind to be in this spaciousness?

MEDITATION EXPERIENCE: CREATING SPACE

In the same way that there is an open sky behind all clouds,
There is a wide-open space behind all sounds.
Can you notice that sound rises and falls
in and out of the bigger space behind it?

This simple technique uses breath awareness and listening. Rather than sitting in a quiet place, try this practice outside or somewhere with environmental noise.

- Sit in a comfortable position on the ground or in a chair, eyes open or closed. Pause for a few exhales and notice where your body meets support.

- Imagine a bathtub filled with water. When you unplug the tub, the water level drains down steadily. Imagine your body is like the tub, and all the heaviness in you drains like water into the ground. Emptying from your head, neck, and shoulders, and down from your arms and torso. Down from your belly into your seat and legs, and then down into the ground.

- Bring your attention to your breath. Notice how each breath rises and falls, in and out of your body, on its own. With your mind, follow the breath's path as it comes in from the *space around you* and as it flows back out into that space. Trace the path of your breath for a minute.

- Shift your attention to the sound of your breath. Listen to the sound that your breath makes as it comes and goes.

- Expand your attention to include the sounds in your immediate surroundings. Notice that, just like your breath, sounds rise and fall.
- Slowly expand your awareness a little at a time. Listen to the sounds of the world rising and falling. Maybe you hear birds, neighbors laughing, traffic. Allow whatever you *notice* to come and go, in and out of your awareness. Just like your breath, sounds come and go, in and out of space. No single sound will stay the same for long. Even a jackhammer will eventually stop.

Let the sounds rise and fall.
Then, just like your breath, and just like the sounds,
let your thoughts and feelings
rise and fall, in and out of this space.
This space is big enough to hold all things.

- Sit for 5 to 20 minutes simply listening to sounds while also noticing how your breath rises and falls on its own.
- To close, pause and welcome yourself into your seat. Set an intention to stay present with yourself as you move out of the meditation.

We are simply training ourselves in being
open and receptive so that we can learn to see
that all things—all thoughts, emotions,
sensations, sounds—will rise and fall in and
out of a larger space.

Yoga Experience:
Standing Flowing Twist

In this flowing yoga exercise, we synchronize our movement with our breath. As we exhale, we twist, compressing our organs; and as we inhale, we return to neutral, making more room for the breath to fill us.

- Begin in Mountain pose.
- Firm the bottom of your seat and upper thighs, hugging them toward your bones to create extra support.
- On your inhale, sweep your arms up; palms meet above your head.
- On your exhale, twist to the right as you open your arms into the shape of a T. Stretch your arms away from each other.
- When your inhale flows back into you, sweep up, and let the breath bring you center again, palms up to the sky.
- Exhale, twist to the other side. Inhale, sweep back up as you come to center.
- After 5 to 10 breaths of twisting, pause. Come back to Mountain.
- Bring a hand to your belly and a hand to your heart. Feel your breath moving in the space under your hands. Follow your next three breaths: Follow each inhale as it comes in from the space around you. Follow each exhale as it flows back out from the space inside you. Mindfully transition into your next moment.

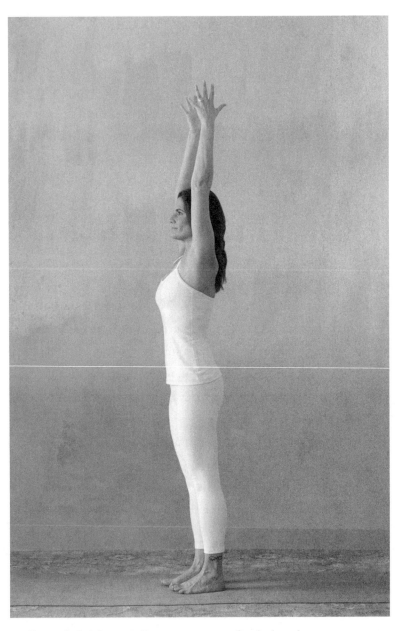

A. *Your inhale lifts you taller, creating space for the breath.*

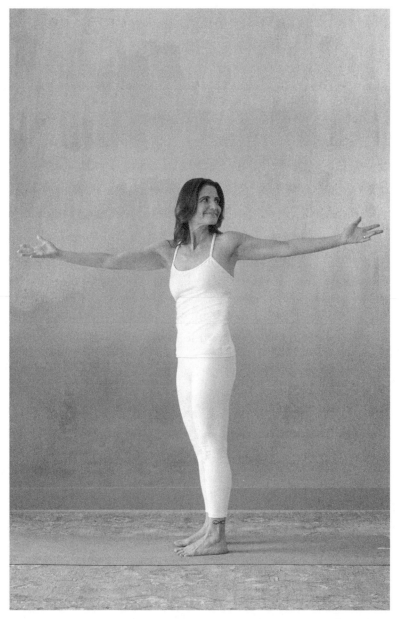

B. *On each exhale, collarbones broaden toward the shoulders as you grow wide.*

Restorative Yoga Experience: Full Relaxation

PROPS: One short-roll blanket. Two blocks. Optional: A blanket for warmth and/or a blanket over your mat for extra cushioning. Two small towels for head and neck support.

SET UP

To begin, set two blocks side by side at the foot of your mat and place your short-roll blanket on top of them. This will go underneath the pit of your knees to help relieve excess tension in your lower back, psoas muscles, and belly as well as along the length of your spine. Have your neck and head support nearby, and also your blanket for warmth.

- Sit facing your rolled blanket. Slowly lower yourself to the floor. Mindfully take your legs over the roll. Bring your legs

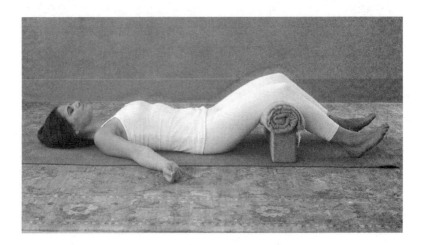

hip-distance apart. If you have an extra blanket, place it over your pelvis and belly, or over your whole body.

- If you need head support, place a rolled towel under your neck along with a folded towel under your head.
- Rest your arms by your sides, either palms down (calming) or palms up (expanding). You may prefer to rest your hands on your belly, with elbows on the floor.

EXPERIENCE FULL RELAXATION

- Take a moment to make adjustments to ensure you are evenly laid out and comfortable. Take several long breaths as you progressively release all of your body weight down onto the ground.
- *Relaxmore* for the next 5 to 20 minutes.
- Before you close your practice, bring your hands to your belly and feel your palms receive your breath. Imagine the breath softening and loosening any lingering hardness inside.
- When you are ready to close, begin to move any way that feels good. Then slowly bring your knees in toward your belly and roll onto your side, making a pillow out of the arm under your head. Relax onto your side completely for a minute.
- Mindfully press up to a comfortable seat to close your practice.

Relaxmore
Make Space and Relax More

Let your body land completely.

Feel the earth receiving you.

Your heels held completely.

Your legs and pelvis dropping into the ground.

Your back spreading across the floor.

The ground welcoming your upper back, shoulders, and head.

The ground will carry you, entirely.

The ground longs to carry you, so your breath can fill you.

Let your breath flow freely in your body.

Welcome your breath into your body.

Imagine the path of your breath—the flow of the breath as it moves

from outside your body into you. And from inside you back out.

Feel where your body meets the space around you.

Imagine the *boundless* space around you that goes on and on.

Let yourself rest in this space that goes on and on.

Feel where your body meets the air.

Feel your skin, a pliable and porous outline, opening to the air.

Imagine you could breathe through your skin.

Allow your outline to soften.

Let your whole being expand into the space around you.

You're bigger than you think you are.

Bring your awareness back to the ground.
Bring your mind through your body.
Imagine there is space for you to expand inside your body.
Imagine the space between your brows expanding.
The space between your ears widening.
Your whole head spacious.
Let your head rest on the ground.

Imagine space inside your shoulders.
Space inside your arms and hands.
Imagine the *volume* inside your hands and fingers.
Feel your arms held by the ground.

Imagine the space between your breastbone and the ground.
Let your breath fill your chest.

Imagine the space between your navel and the ground.
Let your breath expand inside your welcoming belly.
Imagine the space inside your pelvis and legs.
Feel your pelvis and legs on the ground.

Let your entire body be held up by the earth.
Let your breath rise and fall,
in and out of the space that you are.
You are bigger than you think you are.

JOURNALING PROMPTS:
CREATE SPACIOUSNESS

What does being spacious mean to you?

Can you think of a time when you did not feel spacious? Where you felt very tight, limited, closed in?

Can you remember a situation where you alleviated the feeling of being stuck or limited, small or closed in? How did you transform the feeling?

How can you help yourself remember to pause and expand more often?

INSTANT PAUSE AND RESET:
OPEN SKY

U se this Reset while looking at an open sky.

- Stand outside or in front of a window, or gaze at a photograph that features an expansive sky.
- Pause and sense where your body meets the ground. Soften excess gripping in your face, neck, and shoulders. Feel yourself landing completely.
- As you bring your attention to the flow of your breath, gaze into the openness of the sky.
- Follow your next three breaths as they come in from the space around you and expand into your body. Follow them as they move from the space inside you back out into the world around you.
- Notice the continuum of your breathing flowing from outside and inside out.
- Feel how your breath connects you to the space around you.
- To finish, notice your feet on the floor and imagine your head—and your heart—in the shape of the sky. Move into your next moment grounded and open.

CHAPTER SIX

Listening Softly

What is soft is strong.

—LAO TZU

MEETING OUR DEEPER KNOTS

For a long time, my yoga practice was all about getting stronger. I pushed myself to improve my headstands and perfect my Wheel pose. And in every class, I kept expecting my teacher to come over to my mat and tell me what a good job I was doing.

But he didn't.

I expected him to applaud or cheerlead me. But he didn't.

In fact, most of the time, he didn't acknowledge me at all.

I remember thinking, "Why is he not paying attention to how hard I'm working?" I was frustrated and annoyed that I wasn't being recognized for my efforts, but at the same time I felt embarrassed and ashamed about how much I wanted to be "seen" by him.

One day, after working hard on what I hoped would be a flawless Wheel, I relaxed on my mat and was able to notice, just for a moment, how much I was *always* pushing in this class and how much approval I always craved here.

For a moment, I was able to sit with the anger and frustration and embarrassment and shame I felt about wishing my teacher paid more attention to me *without* doing what I usually did: assume I must not be working hard enough and immediately try to figure out what more I should be doing. On this day, instead of starting that old familiar conversation in my head, I simply noticed all the feelings that were emerging up inside me.

As I listened quietly to all my knotted feelings, rather than thinking I had to fix something, I decided (as I'd practiced in meditation) to just let them all *be*. And out of that quiet arose an insight:

- Maybe, possibly, my constant overstriving is not just happening here, on my mat.
- Maybe, possibly, I'm doing excessive work everywhere in my life.
- Maybe, possibly, all these reactions I'm having right now are really about some deeper longing.
- And maybe, possibly, that's something I need to pay attention to.

Because "achieving" had always come so easily to me, the idea that I lived a life of overstriving never really occurred to me before. And on this day, I did not zip away from that idea or add on to it. I simply paused and took it in, the way I would receive a dear friend.

Listening to what arose during my stillness that day not only set me on a new path in my practice, it changed the course of my life.

———

Our body responds

to *everything* we perceive—

everything we take in from outside

and everything we experience

and imagine from within.

DEVELOPING A LISTENING PRACTICE

When we begin to relax, it's not unusual for information to start bubbling up—often in the form of old feelings that our tension is trying to protect us from. So once we begin to release our tension and unfurl those knots, how do we *listen* to what we've stored inside us? How do we meet our "salt"?

A *listening practice* begins with making a choice to relax with whatever comes up in our body, mind, and heart. It means choosing to receive in a tender, nonjudgmental way whatever our tension has been protecting. It means opening up, over and over, to anything we discover, without feeling the need to critique or fix or change.

The mind-set we cultivate to meet ourselves in this way might be the most valuable skill we ever develop. Whether we're breathing into our tight shoulders or sobbing on our yoga mat, the *way* we listen to what our body is saying will either leave us feeling as though we are being cared for or as if we need to protect ourselves. It is our manner and attitude that will leave us feeling open and soft or hardened and closed.

LISTENING WITH OUR HEART

Many mindfulness teachers point to the Chinese character for listening as an instruction manual for *how* to listen. The character is made up of brushstrokes that represent several elements: At the top are the signs for ear and eye; the sign for undivided attention sits in the middle; and it's all held at the bottom by the symbol for heart.

The character itself directs us to not only hear what's being said but also notice visual cues to better understand the true feelings behind the words. We're reminded to offer our full attention, rather than worry about how we're going to respond. And most important, we're asked to receive everything tenderly and openly, attending to it with care.

This type of kind and curious listening is a *heart practice.* Many of us naturally listen this way to the people we love. But we often need to develop the skill of *compassionate* listening when it comes to the way we listen to ourselves.

Compassionate listening

leaves someone feeling

seen

heard

and loved.

LISTENING KINDLY

When I was pregnant, I'd spend my days teaching yoga, running errands, and getting ready to become a mother. During the busy-ness of my day, I barely noticed the sensations inside me. But the minute I sat down to rest, I would feel Baby William poking my insides.

This comes as no surprise. We notice what's going on inside us most profoundly when we grow still. And since being elbowed from the inside is not usually the most pleasant sensation, sometimes becoming still doesn't feel great.

So what do we do when we're met with something uncomfortable? What happens when we must attend to something that challenges us?

Tara Brach uses a great metaphor to illustrate how we typically meet adversity: Imagine you're on your way somewhere important—maybe a job interview or a first date or a conference at your child's school—and suddenly it starts to rain. You're in a big, crazy downpour and there's no way you can wait it out.

And you don't have an umbrella.

This has happened to me more than once, and I have done exactly what she says many of us do. We get angry at ourselves for not checking the weather forecast. We berate ourselves for not bringing an umbrella. We worry we'll show up looking like a drowned rat. We *add on* to the already challenging rainstorm with thoughts that make us feel worse.

Our inner voices can generate more stress and tension than most of the actual events in our lives. Here's the question: Can we be in the rain without critiquing or judging or regretting or just plain wishing things were different? Can we be in the rain with an attitude of kindness or humor? The truth is, whatever our attitude, we're still going to get wet.

LISTENING WITH CURIOSITY

B aby William's jabs and left hooks left me distracted and sleepless. But they also left me with a sense of wonder. "Is that an elbow, or is that a knee?" I'd think. Or simply, "Wow, what's happening in there?"

Early on, I came to my yoga practice with the opposite attitude. I believed I had everything figured out. I knew what I wanted my Wheel pose to look like, so I spent a lot of time pushing myself around, trying to get my body to bend to my will. I was not curious about what it *felt like* to be in Wheel. All I wanted was to feel accomplished.

As babies, we begin life curious about everything we encounter. Then somewhere along the line, we stop wondering and start deciding. We are taught to label things as good or bad, right or wrong, easy or difficult—in large part so we can keep ourselves safe.

Yoga is not about "assuming" a pose or a posture. It's about discovering how we feel in the pose as we're doing it. This distinction is huge, because we usually show up to yoga—and most everything else—having decided a lot of things before we've even gotten there. What if we came to our practice simply *experiencing* the shape our body takes rather than forcing it into the shape we think it needs to be in?

What if we came to our lives saying, "Is that an elbow, or is that a knee?" or "Wow, I wonder what's happening in there"?

———

Feeling like you have it all figured out
takes you out of the present moment.
Curiosity moves you back in.

IT'S *ALWAYS* SOMETHING . . .

When we choose not to decide beforehand how things should be, or will likely be, or even how we hope they will be, we may have a completely different experience in a rainstorm. When we choose not to beat ourselves up about our forgotten umbrella, but rather *befriend* ourselves and our circumstances, we are making a choice to not shut down and close off but instead to stay open and receptive.

When we can remain curious about what's going on inside us—rather than zipping off to all those other places we're so used to going—we can more easily practice being relaxed *even when the baby is moving.*

But how do we repeatedly relax in the face of *whatever* is going on inside us and around us? This question arises all the time because, unfortunately, it's not as if we can release what we're holding just once or twice and be done with it. We must cultivate the habit of continually welcoming ourselves, getting grounded, breathing into what we notice, and making space for it, knowing that in the next hour, the next day—the next minute—we will invariably find ourselves holding again.

Untangling What's Underneath

Even after my breakthrough about the attention I craved in that yoga class, it took me a long time to begin unraveling my deeper knots—learning to pay kind and gentle attention, over and over, to what was stored in my body and in my heart. I unearthed historic layers that I'd hidden from myself and others, not only about how much approval I wanted but also about some of the deeper fears I had around my relationship with my father—how afraid I was of his anger, how afraid I was to lose him to illness, and how afraid I was of never earning his love.

My panic attack after Lisa died was the first crack in the iceberg that left me feeling shaken and raw, unsure of whether I'd ever feel like my "strong" self again. But it was ultimately the way I softened to myself that allowed me to develop a new kind of strength.

Releasing our tension *requires* softness.

It does not require *knowing* all the answers to whatever may come up. We don't need figure everything out. We just need to give ourselves kind and friendly space to receive not only our first uncomfortable thought or feeling but *every* uncomfortable thought or feeling. If we can trust the ground to support us, we can open more fully to what we discover. It's like allowing our breath to come in. We don't have to *do* anything. We simply need to welcome it.

Our real strength is in our ability to soften and receive.

JUST GET WET

A welcoming attitude allows our body to speak to us. Tenderness invites our body to speak again and again.

We are using our skills to keep the stress response "light switch" off and create the conditions that allow us to be curious and kind. Because when we can meet ourselves with curiosity, we are letting ourselves know that we're *okay* right here, right now. And this allows us to create a bit of space to digest whatever arises.

Staying soft and open not only enables us to truly experience the richness of our lives, it also affects how we show up when it's raining. An attitude of kindness affects how we show up to our next thing and our next thing and our next thing after that. It allows us to listen to others more readily. It allows us to more easily take stock of our feelings before we respond.

Yes, we may show up wet. But we also may discover that we actually *like* the rain.

Water is fluid, soft, and yielding.
But water will wear away rock, which is
rigid and cannot yield. As a rule,
whatever is fluid, soft, and yielding
will overcome whatever is rigid and hard.

—Lao Tzu

Listening Softly

Imagine you could breathe
directly through your heart.
Imagine this is where the air flows
in and out of you.

Let your breath flow freely
in and out
through your heart.
Let your breath soften you.
Uncovering layers of you.
Allowing room for you to unfurl.
All of you.

Your breath tenderly receiving
everything it comes in contact with.
Welcoming your deepest feelings
openly, unwaveringly.
Welcoming all your feelings.
Your joys and your sorrows.

Your breath is a gentle listening space.

Your breath listens wholeheartedly
to all that it meets,
staying with you no matter what arises.
Your breath is always present.
Always listening.

Listen to your infinite breath

as it flows

in and out

of your heart.

Your breath will teach you how to listen.

Listen softly.

Listen to yourself

as your breath listens to you.

Practices for Listening Softly

We are practicing listening to the breath.
Practicing noticing the way our breath tenderly meets
everything it comes into contact with.
We are learning to listen to ourselves,
to be with ourselves,
in the way that our breath is unconditionally there for us.
We are training in releasing the habitual tension in our body and mind,
so that we can expand our attention
and wholeheartedly meet whatever arises in us and around us.

CONTEMPLATION

Imagine a dear one who is a compassionate listener. Maybe a teacher, mentor, or even a spiritual leader (you don't have to know the person but rather simply be able to imagine him or her as a caring listener).

Imagine sitting with this person and sharing something important to you . . . maybe something you are grappling with or striving to work out. Or maybe something you are celebrating or cherishing. Whether you need to share from a heavy heart or a light heart, imagine yourself being received and feeling listened to.

As you imagine this sharing, pay attention to as many details as you can:

Who is listening to you? What is the person's posture? Facial expression? Gestures?

What does it feel like to be you while you are being truly listened to, without judgment?

Imagine that you could listen to another person in this manner. Imagine a moment with someone you may come in contact with today or this week. How could you practice this soft listening with that person?

When you are listening to somebody, completely, attentively, then you are listening not only to the words, but also to the feelings of what is being conveyed, to the whole of it, not part of it.

—Jiddu Krishnamurti

MEDITATION EXPERIENCE:
LISTENING OPENLY, SOFTLY, WHOLLY

This simple technique uses creative imagination, the breath, and bodily sensations to help you listen more openly and receptively.

- Sit in a comfortable position on the floor or in a chair. Close your eyes, if you wish. Take a few long exhales out through your mouth as you notice where your body meets support.
- Imagine you have nostrils on the center of your chest where the breath moves in and out. With your awareness, trace the path of your breath in and out through your chest.
- As your breath comes in, imagine it gently expanding the space in your chest. As your breath flows out, imagine it relaxing any rigidity, untangling any knots.
- Place your right hand on your heart center and stack your left palm on top of your right. Bring your attention under your hands. Feel your breath meeting your hands. Welcome your breath. Stay present with the sound and feeling of your breath.
- Practice listening to your breath openly and curiously as you rest your mind in the space under your hands.
- Continue sitting in this meditation for 5 to 10 minutes.

Let your breath flow freely through your heart center,
softening you as it rises and falls.
Each breath tenderly cares for you as it comes and goes.
Each breath softly meeting your heart space.

Listen.
Just as your breath meets you, meet yourself.
Just as the breath
tenderly receives everything it comes into contact with,
welcome whatever arises in you:
thoughts, feelings, even tension.
Your breath stays with you no matter what unfolds.
Stay with yourself.
Softly meet this moment in you.
Softly welcome the whole of you.
Listen inward
openly,
softly,
wholly.

- To close, bring your hands to prayer in front of your chest, bow your head to your heart, and welcome yourself again into your seat, on the ground. Set an intention to pause throughout the day and listen softly to your breath, to yourself, and to another. Slowly expand your awareness back into the space around you.

YOGA EXPERIENCE:
GECKO ARM FLOWING COBRA

In this practice, we are synchronizing our movement with the breath—practicing moving with our breath while we also let our breath move us.

- Lie on your belly. Stretch your legs long. The centers of your kneecaps rest on the ground. Place your hands just off the sides of your mat in line with your breastbone. Come up onto your fingertips. Elbows point up to the sky and widen away from each other.
- On each inhale, press your pelvis, legs, and fingertips down into the ground as you allow your chest to float up.
- There's no need to overeffort or pull yourself up. Like a balloon, your breath will float you up. Rather than working to come up high, think wide, light, and long.

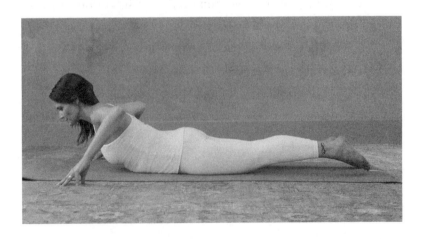

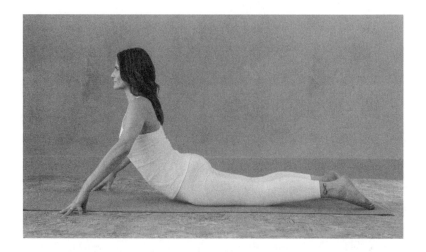

- On each exhalation, lengthen your lower back as you lower down to your mat.
- Repeat 5 to 10 times. Imagine your breath moving in and out through your heart as you flow up and back down in Cobra.
- To finish, pause and rest on your belly for a few moments. Let yourself land completely.
- The main effort in Flowing Cobra is in pressing the pelvis into the ground while gently firming the bottom half of your seat and the backs of your upper thighs. The bottom tips of your shoulder blades gently hug your back. No need to grip your neck or scrunch your shoulders up. Allow all four sides of the neck to be at ease and equal in length.

Restorative Yoga Experience: Easy Fish Pose

This gentle chest-opening pose is a bit more invigorating than our other restorative poses. You may feel gently stimulated as we make room for the breath to expand in the *heart center*.

PROPS: Two short-roll blankets. Two blocks. If you'd like, place a blanket over you for warmth or weight.

SET UP

- Prepare support for your back. Place one short-roll blanket across the middle of your mat. Open it up until the edges touch the back edge of your mat, decreasing the size of your roll.
- Prepare support for your legs. Place two blocks across the front of your mat, with a few inches of space between them. Lay the second short-roll blanket on top of the blocks.
- Sit facing your leg support with your knees bent and feet on the floor. Slowly lie down, positioning yourself so that the blanket roll is just below your armpits, the upper back and head landing on the single layer of unrolled blanket. You will feel the bottom tips of your shoulders up on the roll. Place your arms on the ground just above the rolled blanket, in a T shape or cactus position. Ensure that your neck has a natural cervical curve.
- Mindfully take your legs over the roll. Bring your legs hip-distance apart. Back of your heels should rest on the ground. If you have an extra blanket, place it over your pelvis or over your whole body.

- Make any adjustments you need to ensure that you are evenly laid out and comfortable.

EXPERIENCE FISH

- Take several long breaths and progressively release all your body weight down toward the ground. Let the props hold you up.
- *Relaxmore* for 5 to 10 minutes.
- Before you finish, bring one hand to your belly and one hand to your heart center. Feel your palms receive your breath. *Welcome your caring breath with your caring hands.*
- When you're ready to close, slowly roll onto your right side and enjoy a few quiet breaths. Press to a seated position. Stack your hands over your heart. Feel your breath in your hands. Slowly transition back into the space around you.

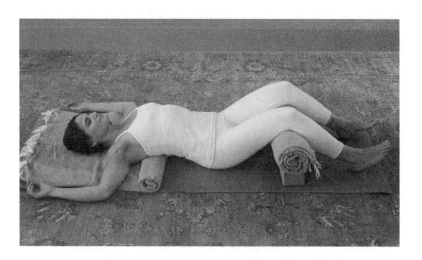

Relaxmore
Listen Softly and Relax More

Let yourself rest on the ground.
No need to hold yourself up.
Let the earth hold you up.

No effort needed.
Effortless legs.
Effortless belly.
Effortless chest.
Effortless arms.
Effortless head.

Allow the earth to receive you.
The ground will hold you
so your breath can fill you.
Let your breath flow freely.

Imagine the breath flowing.
in through the front of your heart
and out through the back of your heart.
Washing through your chest.
Softening you.
Let your heart rest on the ground.

Feel the breath softening you.
Feel the ground holding you
so you can let go more.

———

No work is needed.
Nothing to do.
Nowhere to go.
Let yourself unwind.

Let yourself be held by the ground.
Let yourself be opened by the breath.
Let yourself be held.
Let yourself open.

Let everything be.
Let yourself be.
Let yourself be an

open

soft

listening

space.

JOURNALING PROMPTS: LOVING ATTENTION

Write a letter to yourself proclaiming that you are here to listen to yourself the way a loving friend would listen. Let your body know that you care and that you welcome anything it would like to express. Begin with: *I am here to listen. I will listen openly and with all my heart.*

Ask your body: *How do you feel? What are you carrying? What do you want me to know?*

Then, without overthinking it, put your pen to paper and let your body write you a letter back. Don't write what you think you *should* write . . just let your body speak through your pen as you continually offer yourself compassionate listening. Pause and offer loving attention to whatever shows up on the page.

Instant Pause and Reset: Heart Breathing

E njoy three heart breaths at least three times a day.

- Come to a relaxed position, standing or sitting. Eyes can be open or closed.
- Place a hand over your heart center and feel your breath expanding into your palm. Imagine you have nostrils on your chest where the breath moves in and out. As your breath comes in, imagine it gently expanding your heart space. As your breath flows out, imagine it softening any rigidity.
- Listen to the sound of your breathing as you tune in to the space under your hand.

Listen softly.
Welcome any feelings, thoughts, or sensations you find.
Welcome yourself
into this present moment
as you are.

- After three heart breaths, slowly shift your attention back into the space around you.

CHAPTER SEVEN

Listening Deeply

Between stimulus and response there is a space.
In that space is our power to choose our response.
In our response lies our growth and our freedom.
—VIKTOR E. FRANKL

THE WHISPERING VOICE

About a year before Lisa died, I'd been asked to lead a few yoga sessions at a wellness conference in New York City. This was a great honor; I was a relatively new teacher and I'd only been teaching part-time, but I felt in my heart that this was the work I was truly meant to do.

One day, on one of my hospital visits with Lisa, I brought the conference catalog, planning to share it with her. This was a bold move for me. I usually didn't bring up anything about my career around Lisa. It seemed insensitive to talk about my future when hers was so uncertain. But this time, not only did I share with her my big news, I also confided that, deep down, I'd been considering leaving my corporate job to teach yoga full-time.

There had been a voice inside me urging me to make such a move for a while. A little voice. A whispering voice.

Early on, I had no idea how much credence to give this voice. I loved my job, but also, in my mind, my job was who I *was*. All the foundational ideas I held about myself were validated by my job. Jillian the Achiever. Jillian the Tenacious. Jillian the Succeeder. So why would this voice be suggesting I move on?

I remember telling Lisa all my reservations about leaving my job: I was on a solid career track. I had benefits and vacations and a title and an office. I was good at what I did. It was what I'd always wanted. And it seemed like exactly what I was *supposed to* be doing.

Her response was delivered with a conviction I wasn't expecting; I still hear her words in my head.

"Do what you are called to do," she said.

The more we pause, soften, and listen deeply to what's stored inside us, the easier it becomes to relax our "shoulds" and our "supposed tos." Listening to our inner voice rewires us. It allows us more access to our big-picture thinking, more comfort when we're in a state of "not knowing," and a greater capacity to pause before responding to challenging circumstances in our lives. It becomes easier to feel our own spaciousness and flexibility, allowing us to experience our relationships—and our life—in ways that we were not able to before.

In other words, our perspective begins to change.

HELICOPTER WISDOM

This change in perspective has been described perfectly through a favorite teaching from Erich Schiffmann:

Imagine driving your car on a clear, open highway and up ahead is a tunnel. Everything is going great—smooth sailing—but what you don't know is that once you get into the tunnel, there's a huge traffic jam. Not only that, but the traffic on the other side of the tunnel is at a standstill, so wherever you're on your way to, this route is going to take you a very long time.

But wait! There's a traffic helicopter flying overhead, reporting from its bird's-eye view, letting you know about trouble spots and alternate routes. The helicopter report offers a much broader, more comprehensive perspective about what's going on around you.

From our vantage point inside the car, we *cannot* see what's happening in the tunnel. We *cannot* know what's going on at the other end. We can't even get the helicopter's report unless we tune to the right radio station, to the right frequency.

The helicopter is our wisdom center. It's up there all the time, and its *purpose* is to provide guidance. But if we haven't had enough experience tuning in to its broadcast, we may not know it's there or how helpful it can be. We may pass right by it, tuning instead to some station that's more familiar, one that may not be helpful at all but that we go to all the time.

Deep Listening is the practice of developing a relationship with our wisdom center. We need to feel confident that our helicopter wisdom is always available. Then we need to practice turning on the radio, tuning out the static, and listening in.

THE STATIC OF "NO"

I remember a day, months before I'd shared my conference catalog with Lisa, that I had tried to honor my little inner voice. On a Friday afternoon, I walked into my boss's office and handed him my resignation. Over the weekend, instead of celebrating, I spiraled out. "Oh, no! What have I done? If I don't have a 'title,' how will people know who I am? Without this job, who will I *be*?"

That Monday, I asked for my job back.

This *uh-oh* phenomenon is typical, as its roots are in our "primitive" brain. We are *neurologically* programmed to hear "no" more easily than we can hear "yes," so it can often feel more "important" or more "true."

Of course, there are times where we will need to heed "no." Historically, "no" has probably kept us safe. As a species, "no" has probably even kept us alive. But we need to understand that our wisdom can sometimes be clouded by the "static" of "no."

People generally see what they look for

and hear what they listen for.

—Harper Lee

THE SPACE BETWEEN THE NOTES

We also need to understand that even if we do hear our inner wisdom clearly, we may not yet know that we can trust it. Our wisdom rarely lives in those negative *repeat thoughts* running through our head all day long. Rather, our wisdom arises in the space between those thoughts.

Artur Schnabel, the brilliant classical pianist, was once asked how he plays so beautifully. "The notes I handle no better than many pianists," he reportedly explained. "But the pauses between the notes—ah, that is where the art resides."

Most of us are trained to pay attention only to our "notes"— our thoughts, feelings, circumstances, or even the many things we're so busy "doing" all the time. We get ourselves from one note to another, sometimes effortlessly, and yet we still don't have a relationship with the part of us where our wisdom lives. We simply have not been taught how to pause and notice what is happening inside us regularly enough that we know how to trust the insight we receive.

The good news is that yoga offers us all the opportunity to explore and become familiar with those in-between moments and to practice listening within. The better news is that paying kind and curious attention to the spaces between our "notes" is something we can start doing right away.

The Art of a Mindful Yoga Practice

To become more confident in responding in ways that are wise for us, we simply begin by wondering, "What does it *feel* like to be me right now?" And a mindful yoga practice provides us with all the tools we need to ask that question again and again.

A mindful yoga practice does not focus solely on the poses themselves. Rather, it allows us to pay attention to our bodies the way Schnabel paid attention to the pauses between his notes. It allows us to feel what we are doing, *as* we are doing it, while learning to tune in to the in-the-moment guidance that our wise self provides. It trains us in developing curiosity and remaining open to what we hear.

A mindful practice asks us not to simply execute a pose but to connect with ourselves. First, we need to discover what we feel. Not what we *think* we feel. What we *actually* feel.

What do I feel inside when I'm in this pose?

Where am I resisting?

Where am I overefforting?

Do I need to become more still?

Do I need to engage more?

Is it time to release?

How will I transition from this moment to the next?

How might I take into account the whole of what I'm experiencing in this moment and respond wisely?

A mindful yoga practice allows us to discover what we need to *know* as we need to know it. Our wisdom is already there and always available, but to receive it, we have to open our awareness to the spaces in which it resides. Listening to ourselves with kindness and curiosity not only clears the static, it helps us generate faith in what we hear and our ability to respond.

We practice trusting our inner voice and responding on our mat, so we can listen, trust, and respond with wisdom in our lives.

The more relaxed we are

the more comfortable we become

at spending time in the space

between stimulus and response.

"HOW DO YOU FEEL TODAY?"

I begin every class I teach and every workshop I lead by asking my students, "How are you?"

Usually people smile. Some say, "Good." But I let the question seep into the room. This question sounds like a pleasantry, but it's where we need to begin.

Then I ask, "How do you feel *right now*?"

The room stays quiet for a time, and almost without exception I can see people begin to hold their breath. They freeze a little bit. *How do I feel right now?* They're not accustomed to asking that of themselves.

A few people will usually share with me problems they're having. They tell me which parts of their body hurt. They tell me how stressed they are. How tired. How busy. And we all listen.

Once a few people have spoken, others start to see how they are not alone in their problems. They see how we all feel similarly much of the time. When we all begin to feel more connected, everyone feels safer in the space. And that's when things start to change. The energy in the room shifts, and everyone can feel it.

"What do I need to know?" I'll say, posing a question I've embraced from my years of study with Erich Schiffmann. As a group, we're now ready for this bigger question. Someone might share about some deeper pain, and we all listen with our hearts.

Then, invariably, someone will say how happy he is to be there, an offering that's often scarier than the sharing of sadness. Most of us are used to complaining together, but it's not as typical for us to share our joy.

This first positive remark warms the room, and someone may then talk about her delicious breakfast. Or how excited she is that it's finally spring. It takes a few minutes, but soon we all become less riveted by our problems.

This little evolution occurs every time I lead a workshop. Every time.

And that's important, because it directly parallels what's going on inside us individually whenever we sit to listen to ourselves.

We start off a little tight and frozen.

We need to find our breath.

We need to feel grounded and safe so we can relax into the present moment, because it is only *here* that we can answer these questions:

> *How am I?*
>
> *How do I feel right now?*
>
> *What do I need to know?*

At first, all our problems may arise. All our "shoulds." All our "have tos." All the ways we protect ourselves. All the ways we are not spacious.

We practice welcoming *every part of us* here, even if some parts feel broken or alone.

We practice allowing our breath to center us so we feel safe. So we experience ourselves belonging right here—right now—just as we are.

And we practice doing that again and again, until we can begin to hear and trust the voice inside us that knows how to hold and heal us.

We make space inside ourselves,

so that *being* can speak.

—Martin Heidegger

OUR FEELINGS CAN BE FLUID

Sometimes it's confusing to listen openly to what arises within us, because at our deepest level of understanding the feelings we are faced with can be complex and even contradictory.

I remember experiencing this profoundly several years ago, when someone very close to me suffered a loss so great I could not imagine how she was able to bear it. At her home after the funeral, I thought, "If that were me, I would just curl up into a ball and cry for the rest of my life."

And she did cry. But she also smiled sometimes. I remember watching her receive people and how, even in her sadness, her face would brighten as someone held her. I remember one moment where she laughed a little, and it became clear to me how naturally feelings of deep pain can coexist with loving feelings of lightness, how some of our most difficult emotions can live side by side with some of our most treasured ones, and how easily and fluidly we are able to move between sorrow and joy. Feelings are not fixed; there's never one single way you "should" feel about anything.

WHAT DO WE NEED TO KNOW?

I now think back on that long-ago yoga class where I was always working so hard to capture the attention of my teacher, and I remember the gift I was given that day: a big-sky view of who I was and what I truly longed for.

Now, every morning when I sit to meditate, I ask myself, "What do I need to know today?"

The power of this question is not in the answer but rather in the asking. It's a curious and gentle question. Its purpose is to open us up to the wisdom inside us. The question itself helps clear our static.

When we can listen to ourselves in a welcoming, embracing way, it shifts how we listen in the world. It serves to align our head and our heart.

SHHH! LISTEN

O ver time, I learned to trust what I would hear inside me. A few months after my conversation with Lisa, I quit my job again, this time for good. But it took a while for me to feel completely okay about the change. I was teaching yoga full-time for 2 years before I could say I was a yoga teacher without adding, "I *used to be* in marketing."

None of us are our roles or our circumstances. Still, it's so easy for many of us to confuse what we *have* or what we *do* with who we *are*. We are not our PhDs; we are not our divorces. My client was not his paraplegia. Lisa was not her cancer.

This had always been clear to me about others, but it took a long time for me to see this about myself.

Listening deeply allows us to broaden our perspective of who we really are.

Eventually it allowed me to see how the true strength of yoga was never about mastering headstands. It was about the courage to embrace my authentic self—a *position* that, for me, was much more challenging.

Listening deeply allowed me to know that I was not my marketing job. I was not my achievements. I was not my anxiety. But most important, I was not the little girl who must tirelessly work to get her father's love.

To listen is to lean in, softly,

with a willingness to be changed

by what we hear.

—Mark Nepo

We Are Bigger Than We Think We Are

As our perspective changes, it's easier to see not only the difference between our experiences and who we are but also that we are all much bigger than our circumstances. Once we can relax in that space between stimulus and response, not only are our options different, *we* are different.

Imagine a life where you knew just how to tune in to your helicopter wisdom. Imagine getting into an argument with a loved one and rather than automatically spiraling into that tirade or that crying jag or that eating binge, or running for another glass of wine, you instead *paused* and gave yourself a moment to breathe. A moment to welcome all your feelings. A moment to feel safe. A moment to really feel your feet on the ground. To take another breath, and another and another, until you felt *okay* enough that you could listen within and receive your helicopter report.

In that space, our possibilities expand. In that pause lies our freedom.

Listening Deeply

Let yourself land.
Let your body land on the ground completely.

Let your breath arrive in your body.
Notice the pause at the end of your exhale.
Your inhale will return to you on its own.

Let yourself pause . . . and relax.
Relax expectations, judgments, shoulds.
Listen . . . beyond the words.
Listen . . . beyond knowing.

Listen deeply.
Listen into the space
at the end of your exhale.

Just like the breath,
when we get out of the way,
wisdom flows through us.

Pause. Soften. Receive.
Feel what is happening.

Wisdom whispers
in this space
between the doing.
What do you need to know right now?

Practices for Listening Deeply

We are training in pausing.
We are learning to pause and relax
so that we can make more room for curiosity, listening, insight.
We are practicing listening rather than reacting.

CONTEMPLATION

Imagine that you are already good at tuning in to your helicopter wisdom. That you can remember to pause, breathe, and listen rather than react habitually. Just imagine.

Now bring to mind a current situation where you are usually triggered and you long for a new way to navigate through your same old story. Perhaps you feel confronted at work or repeatedly pressured in some way throughout your day. Maybe you have an ongoing conflict with a partner or a friend. Or you are tangled in a habit that diminishes your well-being.

Picture a situation that normally brings you tension and imagine yourself noticing it *before* you find yourself in a full-blown reaction.

See yourself, in this situation, pausing to feel your feet on the ground and taking a deep breath. Opening up to the possibilities available to you. Imagine yourself responding in a new way to this same old situation.

MEDITATION EXPERIENCE:
SOFT BELLY BREATHING

Softening resistance and tension in our belly is a primary step
in opening our bodies and minds to our deeper wisdom.

- Sit in a comfortable position on the floor or in a chair. Close your eyes, if you wish. Take a few long breaths. Inhaling through your nose and exhaling through your mouth.
- Let your body land on the ground. Let your breath arrive in your body.
- As your breath flows in, feel it move down into your belly. As your breath flows out, let your belly be effortless.
- On your inhale, think, "soft," allowing your belly to receive your breath.
- On the out breath, think, "belly," letting go of any holding and resistance.
- Inhale: "soft."
- Exhale: "belly."

Each inhale, imagine your belly being cared for by the breath.
Each exhale, let the breath loosen any solidity.
Let your breath make room.
Let thoughts, emotions, sensations
rise and fall
in and out
of a spacious belly.

———

- Since our belly is our emotional center, when we soften it, a variety of feelings, thoughts, images, and memories may bubble up. Welcome all that rises and falls. If you find yourself in conversation with a thought or feeling, simply acknowledge that observation, meet yourself kindly, and draw your mind gently back to the flow of your breath.
- After 5 to 10 minutes, place your hands on your belly. Feel your breath meeting your hands. Little by little, expand your awareness into the space around you.
- Close your practice by setting an intention to stay connected to your breath and your belly as you move slowly out of the meditation.

Yoga Experience: Flowing Warrior 2

The intention behind this flowing version of Warrior 2 is to practice moving mindfully in and out of a traditional Warrior pose. As we move at the pace of the breath, we practice pausing in the space at the end of the exhale. It is in this pause that we have time to tune in to our body, time to feel what we are doing as we are doing it.

- To begin, stand in the middle of your mat, facing the long side of your mat. Extend your arms out to the sides in a T shape.
- Step your feet as wide apart as your wrists, the outer edges of your feet parallel to the short edges of your mat.

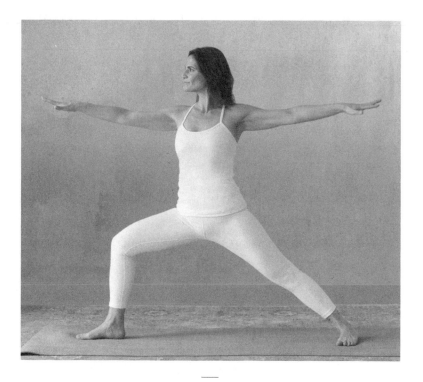

- To come into Warrior 2, leave your left foot as it is and turn your right toes toward the short edge of your mat. If you drew an imaginary line from your right heel, it would intersect roughly at the point of the inner arch of your left foot.
- Bend your right knee, lining it up over your ankle.
- Keep the effort in your legs. Strengthen the backs of your thighs. Firm the bottom half of your seat. Imagine expanding your feet into bigger shoes. Let your breath flow freely in your torso—your ribs free to move with every breath. Grounded, calm, at ease. Strong legs, soft heart.

LET'S FLOW

- On your inhalation, straighten your legs and sweep your arms up to the sky.
- On your exhale, your arms return to the T shape as you lower back into Warrior 2. Pause in the space at the end of each breath.
- Each inhale, push the ground down to come up. Each exhale, let your strong legs lower your light upper body back into Warrior 2.
- Continue to flow 5 to 10 times in and out of Warrior 2. Discover the pace of your breath, as it is happening, and synchronize your movement with your breath.

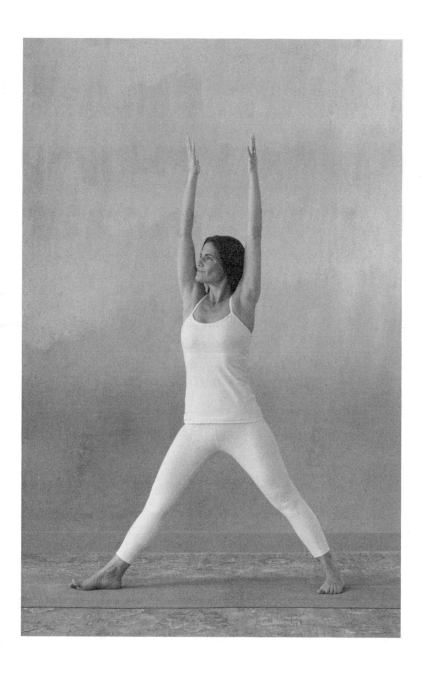

- Pause in Warrior 2 for a few last breaths. Practice listening to your body for insight about how to be in the pose with ease and openness. Ask yourself:

  How can I create a more balanced pose?
  Should I apply more effort? If so, where?
  Should I allow more ease? If so, where?
  Where can I be more stable?
  Where can I be more open?

- Slowly transition to do the other side.

Resist the urge to decide in advance how
you should do any pose or how it should
look or feel. Discover, in the moment,
how to be in the pose, with a balance of
both stability and ease.

Restorative Yoga Experience:
Goddess Pose

PROPS: Two long rectangle–folded blankets stacked. One long-roll blanket. Two blocks. If you'd like, place a blanket over you for warmth.

SET UP

- Prepare support for your back. Place the two stacked blankets vertically up the center of your mat, with about a third of the length hanging off the back of your mat.
- Prepare support for your legs. Sit on your mat, with your blanket stack behind you. Place two blocks across the front of your mat, with a few inches of space between them. Lay the long-roll blanket on top of the blocks.

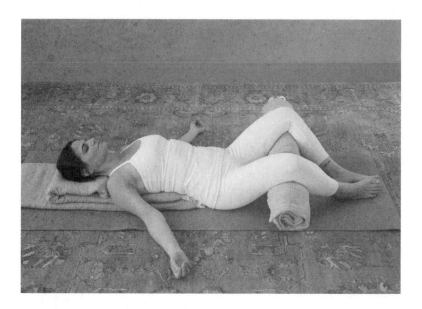

- Bring your legs over the rolled blanket, feet on the floor.
- Lie down. Hold the corners of your blanket stack to help you stay centered as you slowly lower your back down onto the blankets. The blanket stack should fill in the curve of your lower back all the way up to your head. (Your seat is on the mat, not on your blanket.)
- Create head support, if you'd like. Reach back and fold the top blanket under your head and neck until it meets your shoulders. Ensure that your neck has a natural cervical curve.
- Move legs into a diamond shape. Press the soles of your to feet together as you allow your knees to fall apart. With your hands, draw the back of your thigh muscles and flesh wide. Let your outer thighs and knees rest heavily on the rolled blanket.
- Bring your arms by your sides, palms down or palms up. Or rest your hands on your belly, elbows on the ground.
- Make any adjustments you need to ensure that you are evenly laid out, supported, and comfortable.

EXPERIENCE GODDESS POSE

- Slowly scan your awareness down the back of your body. Sense all the places you feel your body making contact with the ground and with the props. Take several long breaths and progressively release all your body weight down toward the ground. Let the props hold you up.
- On your inhale, mentally think, "soft," allowing your belly to receive your breath.

- On your exhale, mentally think, "belly," letting go of any holding and resistance.
- Inhale: "soft." Imagine your belly being cared for by the breath.
- Exhale: "belly." Imagine the breath unraveling any lingering knots inside.
- *Relax more* for 5 to 15 minutes.
- Before you finish, bring your hands to your belly and feel your palms receive your breath. *Welcome your caring breath with your caring hands.*
- When you're ready to close, slowly take your time to roll onto your right side and enjoy a few quiet breaths.
- Take care of yourself as you press to a finishing seated position. Stack your hands over your heart. Feel your breath in your hands. Slowly transition back into the space around you.

Relaxmore
Listen Deeply and Relax More

Let your body land on the ground.

No need to hold yourself up.

Let the earth receive you.

Legs *held* completely by the ground.

Let your seat *land* heavily on the floor.

Your upper back, shoulders, and head releasing into the blankets.

The ground will carry you.

The ground longs to carry you,

so your breath can fill you.

Let your breath arrive in your body.

Let your breath flow freely.

Let your breath be received by a softening belly.

Let your breath gently find

any clinching or any barriers.

Let your breath soften any tension it meets.

Nothing to resist.

Nothing to do.

Your breath will soften you.

Your breath will care for you.

Relax with all that rises and falls.

Relax *more.*

———

Relax and receive your breath.
Let the waves of your breath
rise and fall.
Belly rising and falling
with the breath.
Liquid belly.

Let everything rise and fall on its own.

Relax . . . Listen.
What do you need to know right now?

JOURNALING PROMPTS:
OPEN TO RECEIVE

This journaling practice is a listening practice. To prepare to listen, we will take a few moments to get centered, grounded, and open.

You can use a few elevator breaths (pages 18 to 19) or hourglass breaths (page 39) to lower your weight into your seat. As you grow grounded, expand your awareness to your breath.

Follow the rise and fall of your breath. Let your awareness pause in the open space at the end of the exhale. Allow the breath to flow back to you on its own.

Now imagine you are a big satellite dish, just waiting to receive. Get grounded, tune in, and stay open. Relax and listen with your wide-range pickup capacity.

Ask yourself: *"What do I need to know right now?"*

Put your pen to the page and receive your news.

———

Listen to the wind, it talks.

Listen to the silence, it speaks.

Listen to your heart, it knows.

—Native American proverb

Instant Pause and Reset:
Open, Listen, Choose

Use this Pause and Reset several times a day to relax, listen, and mindfully choose your next action or response.

- Come to a relaxed seated or standing position. Eyes can be open or closed.
- Take a moment to pause. Let your body weight drain down to the ground. Let your breath arrive in your body.
- On your inhale, mentally say, "I am . . ."
- On the out breath, mentally say, "wide open."

Notice the tiny moment of space at the end of each exhale.
Imagine this brief moment as the space between musical notes,
or the white space of a page before any writing takes place.
In this space, relax more.
Listen deeply.

- After your third breath, remind yourself that you can move into the next moment as you choose to.
- Slowly, mindfully, reenter the space around you.

CHAPTER EIGHT

Listening Bravely

The healer you have been looking for

is your own courage

to know

and love

yourself completely.

—YUNG PUEBLO

THE PRINCESS AND THE DRAGON

Once upon a time, there was a rich king and queen who ruled a magnificent kingdom. They had an enchanting daughter, the princess, who was known for her grace and compassion.

Hard times fell upon the king and queen. With no resources left, they arranged for the princess to marry a scaly dragon in exchange for gold.

The princess knew she had to help her parents, but she was afraid of the dragon. So she sought the guidance of the wisest elder woman in the kingdom.

On her wedding night, after the ceremony, the dragon told

the princess it was time to consummate their marriage.

"Yes, Dear Dragon," said the princess, as the wise woman had instructed. "I am ready. But for each article of clothing I remove, you, in turn, must remove a layer of scales."

The dragon was reluctant at first, but his deep longing for the princess moved him to agree.

The princess nervously took off her gown. The dragon skeptically removed some scales.

Under the first gown, the princess wore a second. And when she took that one off, the dragon removed another layer of scales. As each layer was shed, the dragon became slightly more vulnerable and slightly less scary.

The wise woman had directed the princess to dress in so many layers that in order to keep up, the dragon was eventually removing underscales that were so old and so deep he didn't even realize they were there.

Finally, the princess took off her last gown. And the dragon, despite the pain of stripping off his very skin, dug in to remove his last layer. He looked into the eyes of the princess, howling as he pulled away what remained of his armor, and, with that, was transformed into a radiant prince.

The Real Love Story

This is one of my favorite stories for teaching compassion. In this fable, we are the princess and we are *also* the dragon. We are the fair maiden full of goodness and light, and we are *also* the scaly creature who seems ugly and unlovable. Both characters are alive within us.

Our "princess" may be a wellspring of compassion, but she's scared of the dragon. She wishes it would go away. She goes to the wise woman—our wisdom center—secretly hoping she will be told how to get rid of him.

But that's not what happens. The instruction is to accept the dragon, and to slowly and gently lead him through the process of shedding his layers. To stick with him—even though it's scary, even though she doesn't know how things will turn out.

Our deepest wisdom knows that what we need in order to evolve is our own unrelenting kindness toward our "ugly" parts. Our deepest wisdom knows that we need to feel safe and welcomed if we are to uncover what is beneath our protective scales.

The fable directs us to listen deeply, trust, and act.

Our dragon self may seem ugly and scary, but we are being asked to engage with him anyway. We are being reminded that, deep down, our dragon self longs to feel more connected and loved. We all have an unconscious desire to be more integrated and authentic. We all experience an inner pull to marry the various parts of us. Even though we might not always be aware of it, we are all pulled by the promise of wholeness.

What most of us don't realize is that the feelings of love and connectedness we long for are available to us, right here, right now. We can begin to bring them into our lives at any moment.

You, yourself, as much as anybody in the entire universe, deserve your love and affection.

—Buddha

REMOVING OUR SCALES

Metta meditation is an ancient Buddhist practice used to consciously and tenderly create the conditions in which we can experience connectedness. The word *metta* is often translated as "loving-kindness." It is a practice that grows our compassion.

We begin the mediation by bringing a person we love to mind, visualizing them sitting before us, and offering them a metta blessing, such as:

> *May you be happy and at ease.*
> *May you be safe and well.*
> *May you feel loving and loved.*

This seems simple enough—most of us have someone in our life whom we would happily wish all those things for. Someone we're grateful to. Someone we want nothing other than the best for. It's easy to be compassionate toward someone we already love.

But metta does not stop there.

In this practice, we not only bless those closest to us, we also hold in our mind someone we may not know well but whom we appreciate—like the mail carrier or the local barista or that sweet crossing guard. We then bless this person *in the same way* that we bless someone dear to us. Even that step is still pretty easy.

Then we bring to mind someone we find challenging. Someone with whom we could have a good relationship *if only they would remove all their scales.*

We hold the vision of this challenging person in our mind as we consciously offer this person these same blessings. And here's the tricky part: We practice doing this whether we think the person deserves the blessings or not.

My First Metta

The first time I ever did a metta meditation was during a retreat in 1996. I had been meditating for a while by then, so I thought I was all ready for it.

When we were asked us to bring to mind our challenging person, I had no trouble conjuring up my father. I offered him blessings, and yes, it was difficult. I was angry and disappointed and believed that *if only he were different*, we would have had the relationship I longed for.

Then, after we blessed our challenging person, we were asked to offer the metta blessings to ourselves. I had expected blessing my father would be hard. After all, I'd had a lifetime of complicated feelings toward him. But what I discovered that day was that the trickiest person to sit face-to-face with during metta was, by far, myself.

We do not practice cultivating a tender, accepting, curious attitude toward ourselves simply so that we can speak to ourselves in a kinder voice—although that is a good, solid benefit of metta. We practice cultivating this softness so we can offer love to ourselves. And just as important: so that we can receive it.

The first time I attempted to offer myself blessings, I was not expecting to feel so resistant. I was not prepared for how undeserving I'd feel. I was certainly not expecting to cry. Initially, I couldn't offer or accept the blessing at all, and to get through the meditation, I had to pretend that my best friend was the one blessing me.

By comparison, offering loving-kindness to my father was a walk in the park.

When we practice metta,

it affects how we feel toward ourselves.

And how we feel toward ourselves

affects how we feel about others.

Bravely Removing Our Barriers

The dragon from our fable lives with scales that he's come by honestly, as we all do. We're designed to protect ourselves when we feel threatened or vulnerable. We armor ourselves because somewhere along the line, something made us feel unsafe. It can happen without our being aware of it. It may have been something we experienced directly or it may even be something our parents or grandparents experienced. It doesn't matter where our scales come from. What matters is that inside we feel at risk of being slayed.

But what matters more is that we recognize the scales that protect us are also the barriers that exist between ourselves and the deep connections we long for. They're barriers we put up against receiving our breath, against giving and receiving love, against experiencing our wholeness.

Removing layers of scales is an act of courage. Writer Doris Lessing summed it up in this way: "Almost all humans . . . have strange imaginings. The strangest of these is a belief that they can progress only by improvement. Those who understand will realize that we are much more in need of stripping off than adding on."

Our work is to learn how to remove our barriers. Our work is to tenderly stop resisting. Our work is to lovingly strip away our scales.

May you be happy and at ease.
May you be safe and well.
May you feel loving and loved.

We offer this blessing because doing so makes *our* barriers more porous. We are not waiting until someone deserves the blessing. We are offering it freely, which expands our capacity to feel our compassion and our connectedness.

We are *already* whole, we are *already* connected, we are *already* complete.

Feeling safe and relaxed while saying these words *is* what soft-
ens us. It allows us to experience the love inside us and around us,
right now.

It doesn't matter how long we may have been

stuck in a sense of our limitations.

If we go into a darkened room and turn on

the light, it doesn't matter if the room has

been dark for a day, a week, or ten thousand

years—we turn on the light and it is illuminated.

Once we control our capacity for love and

happiness, the light has been turned on.

—Sharon Salzberg

BLOOMING ANYWAY

Metta trains us to stay open in front of our "triggers." We
practice breathing and relaxing with our uncomfortable
relationships, because if we can meet our most challenging people in our head and still feel *okay*, we become better at doing it in
real life.

Metta is not a practice where we *replace* negative feelings with positive ones. We're not trying to change the person we're calling to mind. We're noticing how and when and where we close down in reaction to what's in front of us. We're learning how to be sad and hurt and angry and still feel connected to our own love.

We're practicing staying open on purpose, choosing to soften no matter how we feel.

We don't do this for the benefit of that challenging person. We do it for ourselves. Because when we're tense and shut down in our body and in our heart, we cannot feel our wholeness.

It's like a flower whose sweet scent wafts out into the world. The flower doesn't minimize itself depending on who walks by—radiating beauty and splendor for worthy people and shutting itself down for the unworthy. Flowers emit their scent for everyone.

We were all meant to radiate.

And then the day came

When the risk to remain tight in a bud

Became more painful

Than the risk it took to blossom.

—Elizabeth Appell

You Say You Want an Evolution

Compassion begets compassion. When someone is treated with kindness and compassion, they are more apt to act kindly themselves. But also, when we consciously choose compassion toward another, we're actually flexing our "empathy muscle" and making it stronger.

When we feel compassion, we release hormones that make it easier to see our similarities, as opposed to the stress hormones that can keep us focused on our differences. Our "compassion hormones" make it easier to be grateful rather than cynical. We naturally begin to relax some of the ways we guard ourselves. We perceive fewer boundaries between ourselves and the rest of the world, and this makes us feel that we're part of something much bigger.

In her blog, *Velveteen Rabbi*, Rachel Barenblat recounts a story from spiritual teacher Rabbi Jeff Roth: "Two waves are hanging out together in the sea, a big wave and a little wave. And the big wave is anxious and scared. The little wave says, 'Why are you so afraid?' And the big wave says, 'If you could see what I see, you'd be afraid, too. Up ahead of us there are some cliffs, and I can see where we're going—every wave in front of us goes up to those cliffs, and smashes into them, and disappears.'

"And the little wave smiles and says, 'If you could see what I see, you wouldn't be afraid.' And the big wave asks, 'What's that?' And the little wave says, 'We're not waves—we're water.'"

A compassion practice helps us feel our inherent connectedness. A compassion practice helps us understand that we do not need our circumstances to be "just so" in order to feel connected, loving, vibrant, and alive. It's as if we're able to see the world—the same world we've always lived in—through an entirely different set of eyes.

DIFFERENTLY EVER AFTER

At the end of our story, the princess and the dragon were connected in a way they were unable to be before. This is how we come to our wholeness: by softly and tenderly releasing whatever we hold or cling to that keeps us separate from our true selves.

When I was able to give gentle attention to my many layers of protection, my scales softened. Some of them fell away. And as I learned to befriend myself and receive my own love, I began to experience my father differently.

Once I no longer needed my father in order to feel validated or loved, I could see how he was vulnerable in his own way. How he, too, was a walking summary of all his undigested pain. As my "container" got bigger, my "salt" became less concentrated and the water less murky. And once I could feel compassion for my father, our relationship did change. Not because *he* had changed. But because I had.

What you do for yourself,

any gesture of kindness,

any gesture of gentleness,

any gesture of honesty and clear seeing

toward yourself

will affect how you experience your world.

In fact, it will transform how you experience

the world.

What you do for yourself, you're doing for

others,

and what you do for others, you're doing for

yourself.

—Pema Chödrön

Listening Bravely

The ground longs to carry you
So your breath can fill you.
Let your body land on the ground.
Let your loving breath fill you.

Feel your breath
meeting you tenderly.
Feel your breath
caring for you inside.

Pause. Relax more.

Feel where your body
meets the space around you.
Feel where your body
meets the air.

Feel your skin
a porous outline
opening to the air.

Imagine you could breathe through your skin.
Imagine that the grace of your breath could flow in and out
directly through your skin.

Porous body.
Porous mind.
Porous heart.

———

Softening
into the wholeness
you already are.

Relax.
Open.
Listen.

You are already whole.
You are *already* whole.
You are already *whole*.

Practices for Listening Bravely

We are learning how relaxing our tension can
help us expand our capacity to feel our compassion
and our connectedness—
to ourselves and others.
We are practicing relaxing and opening when we feel
the impulse to do the opposite.
We are practicing on our mats,
so we can be more open and compassionate
in the daily moments of our life.

CONTEMPLATION

Visualize a blooming flower. It can be the memory of a real flower or one from your imagination. Picture yourself stopping to smell the flower, appreciating its fragrance and beauty. Now imagine another person stopping to enjoy it. And another person, and another.

Notice that the flower doesn't change its nature depending on who is standing in front of it. It doesn't radiate its fragrant beauty and splendor for some people and shut itself down for others. It radiates for everyone.

Now imagine what it would be like to stand in front of someone you feel very loving toward. Imagine being in your body, relaxing in that person's presence. Like a flower, you radiate your true nature. Notice how you feel in your body when you radiate.

Now, can you imagine standing this way—grounded, relaxed, and connected to your heart—with someone slightly challenging? (Don't select someone highly charged; start easy.) What would it be like to be you, relaxing in front of someone you normally shrink from or tighten up in front of? Take a moment to feel your breath and your body while you imagine a new capacity to soften during a time that you would normally harden.

Imagine what it might be like to not diminish your true self, no matter who is walking by.

Your task is not to seek for love,

but merely to seek and find all the barriers

within yourself

that you have built against it.

—Rumi

MEDITATION EXPERIENCE: METTA

Metta meditation is an ancient technique that combines visualization, affirmations, and self-awareness to help release tension and cultivate compassion. Metta expands our ability to offer and receive love.

In this variation of metta, we begin by getting grounded and relaxed. Then we visualize someone sitting before us as we offer them a metta blessing. (We will progressively offer metta to several people with whom we have different relationships.) As we move through the visualizations, we observe ourselves, without judgment, and notice any emotions, thoughts, or sensations that arise. Remember, it's normal for our practices to trigger anything from vivid memories and intense feelings to boredom, indifference, or even numbness. We are training in relaxing with *whatever* we experience. We are learning that we can choose to relax rather than follow the impulse to contract and harden. Ultimately, what we practice in our minds and bodies on purpose can help us return to a state of compassion more naturally in our life. If the phrases I offer in this meditation don't resonate with you, feel free to create your own.

- Sit in a comfortable position on the ground or in a chair. Close your eyes, if you wish. Pause for a few exhales and notice where your body meets support.
- Mentally scan your whole body for habitual tension. No need to clench anywhere in your head, your neck, your shoulders. Let your body weight drain down your torso, down through your belly. Let yourself land on the ground completely.
- Bring to mind someone currently in your life who is easy to love. Someone you are grateful for. Don't worry if more than one person pops up. You can do this several times a week and include many different people. For now, start with one.
- See that person fully in your mind's eye, as if they are sitting

in front of you. Greet them. Welcome them with some sort of caring gesture, anything that feels authentic to you. Imagine you can look directly into their eyes, as you offer these metta phrases—like a wish or a blessing for them. As you say these words in your mind, notice how you feel.

May you be happy and at ease.
May you be safe and well.
May you feel loving.
And may you feel loved.

- Allow this image of your dear one to slowly fade as you take a deep breath and relax.
- Next, bring to mind a person you don't know very well but still feel *generally* friendly toward—your mail carrier, bank teller, someone you see on the bus every day. Imagine this person sitting across from you. Look into their eyes. As you mentally offer them these wishes, notice how you feel.

May you be happy and at ease.
May you be safe and well.
May you feel loving.
And may you feel loved.

- Allow their image to fade as you pause to reground and sense your breath.
- Now bring to mind a person you feel some sort of challenge with. You don't have to choose your most "charged" relationship. It could be someone you can tolerate a bit, but tend to

tighten up around. (Eventually you may choose to explore working with more difficult relationships.) Take a deep breath. Relax again as you picture this person sitting across from you. Look into their eyes. As you mentally offer them these wishes, notice how you feel.

May you be happy and at ease.
May you be safe and well.
May you feel loving.
And may you feel loved.

- Allow this person to slowly fade from your mind's eye and take a few deep breaths.
- Slowly move your attention back toward someone easy to be with. Someone you love. Add a second person you feel good-will toward. Then slowly let a group form in your mind—your book club, PTA, running group, congregation, the people you have lunch with at work. Progressively picture your community, town, state, country, and then the world. See the whole planet in your mind as you mentally offer all beings these wishes. Notice how you feel.

May all beings be happy and at ease.
May all beings be safe and well.
May all beings feel loving.
And may all beings feel loved.

- Pause to feel your breath and be aware that you, too, are on the planet. That you, too, are included in "all beings." That you, too, deserve your love and affection. And now picture yourself sitting across from yourself. Look into your own eyes as if you were looking into a mirror. Notice how you feel as you offer this blessing to yourself.

> *May I be happy and at ease.*
> *May I be safe and well.*
> *May I feel loving.*
> *And may I feel loved.*

- Let this image slowly fade. Feel your body land on the ground. Feel your breath arrive in your body.
- To close, bring one hand to your heart and one to your belly. Feel your breath with your hands. Welcome your breath into your body. Set an intention to stay with your breath, to stay with yourself, as you transition out of the meditation and into your next activity.

If it is difficult to do metta for yourself (as it was for me initially), feel free to imagine someone you love offering you the phrases. Simply practicing receiving love. When that feels possible, then visualize offering it to yourself. Don't worry if it takes time. Love is patient. Be gentle.

YOGA EXPERIENCE:
LOW LUNGE

PROPS: Two blocks. A short rectangle—folded blanket.

SET UP

Place your blocks on either side of the front of your mat in their highest position. If you'd like, place the blanket on your mat to cushion your knees.

- Come onto all fours in a tabletop position, your spine in a neutral position.
- Step your left foot between your hands. Bring your hands to the blocks and slide them back directly under your shoulders so your arms make a vertical line to the floor.
- Your front knee lines up over your ankle, shin vertical to the floor. Your back knee is on the ground.
- Curl the ball of your back foot into the floor and press it down to leave a deep print in your mat. Spread through both footprints equally.
- Continually deepen your footprints in your mat as you *firm* the bottom of your seat and back upper thighs.
- Let your weight drain down out of your upper body and into your pelvis, legs, and feet.
- Release any gripping in your shoulders. Your upper body light. Your crown floats up toward the sky, and the back of your neck is soft and wide. Allow your breath to flow through your body.

- After 5 to 10 breaths, slowly bring your hands to the ground. Gather your belly and come back to all fours. Repeat on the other side.
- To finish, come back to all fours, sit back on your heels, and pause. Feel your connection to the breath and to the space around you.

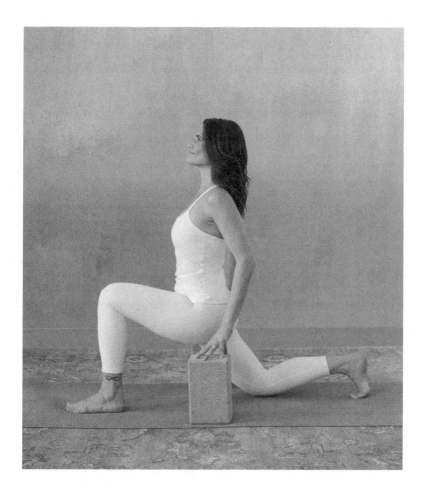

Restorative Yoga Experience: Full Relaxation

PROPS: One short-roll blanket. Two blocks. Optional: A blanket for warmth and/or a blanket over your mat for extra cushion. Two small towels for head and neck support.

SET UP

To begin, set two blocks side by side at the foot of your mat and place your short-roll blanket on top of them. This will go underneath the pit of your knees. Have your neck and head support nearby, and your blanket for warmth.

- Sit facing your rolled blanket. Slowly lower yourself to the floor. Mindfully take your legs over the roll. Bring your legs hip-distance apart. Back of your heels rest on the ground.
- Create head support, if you need it, by placing a rolled towel under your neck along with a folded towel under your head.
- Rest your arms by your sides, either palms down (calming) or palms up (expanding). Or rest your hands on your belly, with elbows on the floor.

EXPERIENCE FULL RELAXATION

- Take a moment to make adjustments to ensure you are evenly laid out and comfortable. Take several long breaths as you progressively release all of your body weight down onto the ground.

- *Relaxmore* for the next 5 to 20 minutes.
- Before you close your practice, bring your hands to your belly and feel your palms receive your breath. Imagine the breath softening and loosening any lingering hardness inside.
- When you are ready to close, begin to move any way that feels good. Then slowly bring your knees in toward your belly and roll onto your side, making a pillow out of the arm under your head. Relax onto your side completely for a minute.
- Take your time to mindfully press up to sitting and close your practice.
- *Relaxmore* for 5 to 10 minutes.

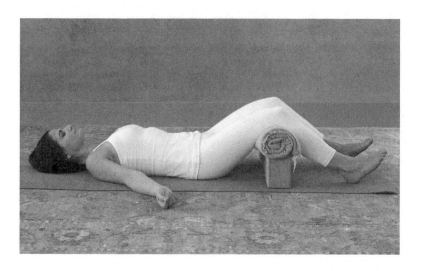

Relaxmore
LISTEN BRAVELY AND RELAX MORE

Let your body land on the ground.
Let the earth receive you.

Your heels held completely.
Your legs and pelvis
dropping into the ground.

Let your upper back, shoulders, and head
rest completely on the ground.
Your back spreading across the floor.
The ground will hold you up.

The ground longs to carry you,
so your breath can fill you.

Welcome your breath
into your body.
Let the waves of breath
flow freely on their own.

Let everything be, as it is.
Nothing to resist.
Nothing to do.

Everything rising and falling.

Feel where your skin meets the air.

Feel your skin,

your porous outline,

opening to the air.

Imagine you could breathe through your skin.

Porous body . . . Porous mind . . . Porous heart.

The infinite breath expands you.

Relax more

and expand into yourself.

You are bigger than you think you are.

You are already whole.

You *are* whole.

Develop a mind so filled with love,

it resembles space . . .

—Buddha

JOURNALING PROMPTS: SUPPORT YOURSELF

Can you recall a time when you unexpectedly received a compassionate response from someone when you really needed it? Write about this in as much detail as you can.

Can you remember a situation where you shifted from feeling shut down and closed-hearted? What do you think helped you transition from tight to tender? Write about it in as much details as you can recall.

How can you encourage yourself to stay open today in those moments when you feel yourself tensing up? How can you encourage yourself to listen bravely today?

Listening is where love begins:
listening to ourselves and then to our
neighbors.
—Fred Rogers (Mr. Rogers)

INSTANT PAUSE AND RESET: METTA EXPANSION

Pause several times a day to notice how you feel, release any accumulated tension, and reconnect to a state of warmth and openness.

- Pause and notice what is going on in your mind and body. Simply take a moment to notice *how you are* and to welcome yourself *as you are.*
- Bring to mind someone easy to love, someone whom you feel grateful toward—even a pet.
- Take three heart breaths as you imagine extending your gratitude and love to this being. Pay attention to how you feel in your body and mind as you extend your gratitude.
- Slowly bring your awareness back to where your buddy meets support, then expand it into the space around you. Allow yourself to stay connected to your breath and your heart space as you move back into your next activity.

CHAPTER NINE

Listening Again and Again and Again

It's not a matter of faith. It's a matter of practice.

—THICH NHAT HANH

VALENTINE'S DAY

My father died on Valentine's Day, 2011.

Throughout much of his life, my dad suffered physical and mental tension, serious illness, and childhood pain. It was hard for him to ever truly feel good, and deep connection to others did not come easily. Yet my practice has allowed me to see that even though it may not have been in the form I needed or wanted, my father loved me the best he was able.

In the years before his death, I could recognize the ways in which my father *had* reached out to me and supported me. And the more I noticed those things, the more they seemed to happen. My dad would call me after seeing a segment about yoga on a morning TV talk show, excited to recount what he'd learned. He'd clip articles about brain research or meditation out of his Florida

---

newspaper and mail them to me in New Jersey. Sometimes when I was visiting, we'd go out on his boat, and instead of insisting we go fishing (his passion), we'd motor around looking for dolphins (my joy).

With his every gesture, I felt more loved. And in turn, I became more soft-hearted in his presence, something I never thought possible.

Today when I bring my dad to mind, I feel great warmth toward him. I see him through eyes of compassion rather than eyes of hurt. I am grateful for this. It allowed me to spend the final years of his life in the kind of relationship I'd always wanted.

This past Valentine's Day, I wanted to write a blog post about how love can transform us, and because it was an anniversary of his passing, I decided to write about my dad. I started bringing to mind stories from my childhood. In one, I was in a big soccer tournament, playing as if my life depended on it. I'd just defended a goal by slide-tackling two boys, and right away I looked to the sidelines, certain my dad would be beaming. But he was not there. He'd apparently walked off to watch my brother practicing on the adjacent field. That moment of disappointment has always been so vivid—a memory that, even as an adult, can make my face feel hot and my throat contract, as if it just happened yesterday.

But this Valentine's Day, I felt none of that. The memory was alive, but the sting was gone.

In fact, I even laughed about how ridiculous it now seems to have thought that taking down soccer players would have made my dad proud. And at the same time, I felt compassion—not only for my father but also for that little girl.

Through this work, much of my "Dad salt" has dissolved. My body doesn't hold those old experiences as "pain" any longer, and neither does my heart. My stories still live inside me, but they no longer own me.

THE WOLF WE FEED

Even if it feels as if they define us, we can always make a choice to evolve our stories. And in doing so, we ourselves evolve.

There's a Native American tale about a grandfather trying to impart this wisdom to his young grandson:

The grandfather explains that it's as if we each have two wolves living within us. One wolf represents all that we consider good: kindness, courage, compassion, love. The other wolf represents the darker parts: fear, hatred, anger, greed.

"The two wolves are in constant battle," the grandfather tells the boy, letting him know that *everyone* struggles with their own conflict between darkness and light.

"Which wolf wins?" the boy asks his grandpa.

"Whichever one you feed."

It is true that I do not feel the sting of my father these days, but this is also true: If I start telling myself my angry and hurt stories over and over, my "Dad salt" becomes concentrated all over again. And sometimes I do slip into those stories. But I now know that what I'm doing is feeding that dark wolf. *I'm* the one choosing which wolf to nourish and make strong.

When we are relaxed we have the capacity
to direct the mind in more healing ways—
which has a further impact on our healing.
—Herbert Benson, MD

Hey! Want a Do-Over?

It's not only the stories of our past that we need to create kind, gentle space for. New salt shows up every single day—as challenges, difficult feelings, tough encounters. Our salt can come from big things or little things; the magnitude of the event is not important. We simply want to be able to pause and recognize it all as salt— then make the choice to relax and to stay present and open.

The good news is, we usually don't have to look too far for opportunities to practice this. For example, when my son was in kindergarten, getting him out the door in the morning for school was an exhausting feat. He had his own ideas about how mornings should go (ideas that were in direct opposition to mine!). It seemed like every day we were in conflict. I felt like I was always yelling.

One day, I had what seemed like a crazy idea: What if I used skills from my practice to help my son through some of his stubborn childhood moments?

The next time William and I disagreed—say, about how much time it should take for a 5-year-old to get dressed and out the door—and emotions started to escalate, rather than yelling, I said, "Hey, want a do-over?"

This is how we pause in real life. We notice the direction our current reactions are taking us. We stop, get grounded, and turn our attention to the breath. We tune in to our wisdom center and give our thoughts and feelings some space. We allow ourselves to *feel* what we feel, but we also remind ourselves to loosen our grip on those feelings, allowing them to rise and fall. And in this spaciousness, we can *choose* whether we want to stay on our familiar route or instead try some new one that may better serve our relationships and our own well-being.

Often, by the time we need a do-over, it can seem as though it's already too late. We might feel like we've dug in so deeply, we *must* stick to our position. Or maybe our "thought conversation" has taken root so solidly, we forget that it will dissipate if we simply don't add on to it. We forget that we always have the ability to change. We forget that we can always begin again.

When I offered William a do-over that day, I wasn't just giving *him* a chance to make a new choice during our tough morning, I was offering that possibility to us both. Pausing was something we both needed, an opportunity we both welcomed. It gave us *both* a chance to evolve.

It is not the strongest of the species that survives, nor the most intelligent, but the one more responsive to change.

—Charles Darwin

This Is How We *Do* It

Not only *can* we offer ourselves a do-over every day, but doing so is truly the essence of what our practice is all about.

At the end of my workshops, I remind my students (again and again) that what we're doing does not have an "end" where everything is "fixed." We all have this idea floating around inside us that once we nail this meditation thing or this yoga thing, our lives will finally be just as we've always hoped they'll be—all our troubles behind us.

We are not trying to create a trouble-free life, even if that were possible. We're trying to create for ourselves the experience of well-being. Not a life that's perfect, but rather a life where we feel *okay* no matter what's going on around us.

I also make the point that learning to relax doesn't mean we surrender or become passive.

I have always wanted to create big, wonderful things in life, and that hasn't changed. What's changed is that I used to create in order to make up for feeling that I was somehow "not enough." I believed I had to always be pushing or chasing after something in order to feel *okay.*

When I practice Deep Listening, I am motivated more than ever to do big things in the world, but that motivation no longer comes from feeling unworthy, as if I need to please everyone or prove myself. Instead, I feel organically drawn toward my goals. It's an experience that leaves me energized and excited, confident and alive.

When we truly feel we're enough *just the way we are in the world*, our creativity springs from a deeper place, where our head and heart are aligned.

Setting Our Own Intentions

For years, I've incorporated the ritual of *intention setting* into the retreats I lead.

"Setting intentions" can sound very New Agey, but it's something most of us already do on a regular basis. For example, New Year's Eve is, for many, a time of ritualistic intention setting. On that night we pause, take a moment to consider our present, and perhaps resolve to step into the future differently.

I love creating rituals, especially for the message it sends: *Slow down. Pay attention. This is important.*

On the last day of each retreat, after we've spent days getting grounded, clear, and open, we pause to set an intention before reentering "real life." I ask each person to put some thought into how he or she wants to walk forward into life and to write it down on a note card. We then stand in a circle around a bonfire. In spiritual ceremonies, fire symbolizes purification and transformation. One by one, we step forward and offer our card to the flames. Together, we create a sacred moment around our desire to evolve.

But setting intentions doesn't *require* a ritual. I set intentions for myself regularly—and few of them involve a bonfire.

I celebrate most holidays (and all my birthdays) reminding myself how I want to walk into my future. What choices I want to make.

I try to begin every class I teach by setting an intention to be present and available to whoever is in the room with me. I ask to be clear so I can listen deeply to what my students have to say. What they have to teach me.

And I ask students in my weekly classes to pause for a moment and consider why they have come today. What do they need from their practice right now? What do they want to cultivate?

If people don't know exactly what they want for themselves in the moment, I suggest an easy, go-to intention that I consider invaluable: "May I be open to whatever I need to know right now."

Whenever I feel as if I'm losing my ability to stay grounded and show up fully, I set an intention to be in the world as my whole, authentic self. I remind myself that I can choose which wolf to feed.

And what's happened in my life is this: I still have tough days. I still feel anger and jealousy, confusion and disappointment. But all those feelings now have a much shorter shelf life. It's easier for me to recognize them before they take hold. It's easier to move through them and back into a state of warmth and openness.

My students report similar experiences. The stress in their lives does not go away. But how they respond to it—and more important, how it affects them—is different.

Setting intentions is part of the process of creating new, more nourishing habits. Doing so helps to diminish old habits that do not support us. The more often we pause and set an intention, the easier it becomes to make wise choices. And then the easier it is to do it again.

The Future Starts Now

There's no need to wait until we are in a heated battle with a loved one to call a do-over, and there's no need to wait for a particular day to start evolving our future. We have all the tools we need to affect our well-being right now. We can start every day with a fresh intention. We can remind ourselves that we want to enter every new moment anchored in the present, with a body that's calm, a mind that's clear, and a heart that's open. Just this reminder not only changes our experience of our today, it plants the seeds for our tomorrow.

In *Your True Home*, Thich Nhat Hahn writes, "We can only take care of the future by taking care of the present moment, because the future is made out of only one substance: the present."

Welcome Back . . . Again and Again and Again

Deep Listening is a lifelong practice. There is no magical moment when we're "done."

We wake up each day, welcome ourselves, and begin again.

Throughout our life, throughout our year, throughout our day, throughout the next hour—we will forget that, like our breath, everything rises and falls. We will forget that our thoughts, our feelings, and our circumstances all rise and fall. We will forget that the nature of everything is to change. That we, too, are meant to change. We will forget that we can be here, right now, simply relaxing with what is.

We will get stressed again. We will trip out again. We will feel separate and alone again. It's not a matter of *if*, it's a matter of *when*.

We *will* get lost again. But we can come back.

We are learning to *remember* that we can come back. We are practicing how to welcome ourselves back. How to pause and begin again.

We practice meeting ourselves softly, kindly, and curiously, over and over, one breath at a time and ask:

"How can I care for myself?"

"How can I accept and love myself, right here and right now, so I can respond to what's going on in front of me in a way that nourishes my life?"

"How can I listen softly, deeply, and bravely to what my heart is saying, so that my authentic self can shine through?"

"How can I show up in a more caring way for the people I love?"

Our practice allows us to set an intention every day to connect with our true self—for comfort, for guidance, for love.

Gently and compassionately, we welcome ourselves back to ourselves. Again and again and again.

Listening Again and Again

Come pause for a moment.
Let your weight drain down
onto the earth.
Let your body land on the ground.

Let yourself receive a few deep breaths.
Feel your breath moving through you.
Moving you.

Ride the waves of your breath
into the present moment.
Let your breath bring you here
now.

It doesn't matter where you've been.
You can come back here
now.
You don't need to do anything.
You don't need to be any way.
You don't need to be "good" or "right."
You only need to be willing
to come back.
To begin again.

This is how we do it.
Over and over again.
We show up kindly and curiously.
We slow down, get grounded, breathe,
We relax and breathe again.
Pause and breathe again.
Release and breathe again
Listen and breathe again
and again.

One breath at a time we arrive.
Even if only for one breath.

One breath at a time
we allow ourselves to be at ease.
Even if only for one breath.

One breath at a time we pause
and listen
softly, deeply, bravely.
Even if only for one breath.

We may hear
our vulnerability
our sadness, our anger
our confusion, our fear.

We may hear
our gratitude
our joy, our prayers
our blessings
our love.

One breath at a time
we listen.

And then
we forget.
We get lost.
We zip away.

That's okay.
We are always welcome back.
We can always begin again.
We can welcome ourselves back
to begin again
and again
and yet
again.

One breath at a time we listen.
We come back.

One breath at a time
we free ourselves to feel whole.

Every time we listen deeply
we can remember our wholeness.
Every time we listen deeply
we can remember our way back.

And every time we listen deeply
we evolve.

Listen deeply.
You will know.

Practices for Listening Again and Again

We are learning how to remind ourselves
that we always have a choice about
how we step into the future.
We are learning to remind ourselves
that we can always
begin again.

CONTEMPLATION

Picture yourself at a time in the past when you were feeling unwell, resisting change, or grieving a loss of some kind. Now imagine that you could go back and be with your past self during this challenging time. Imagine offering kindhearted attention to yourself. Let your past self feel your presence and know that you are listening softly. Listening deeply.

Ask your past self:

How are you?

How do you feel?

Consider that while these old feelings may have originated

because you felt you needed protection at the time, they now may no longer serve you. They now may limit your well-being and happiness. Can you imagine befriending your past self and encouraging a softening around this old story that you carry with you in order to make room for something new to evolve?

Then ask your past self:

Is there anything you'd like to stop holding on to, stop carrying?

By becoming intimate with how we close

down and how we open up,

we awaken our unlimited potential.

—Pema Chödrön

MEDITATION EXPERIENCE: OPEN HANDS, OPEN MIND, OPEN HEART

This is a simple meditation that combines small movements, body awareness, and awareness of the space around you. It will help you reground and open up. It can be done in just a few minutes or extended for as long as you'd like.

- Sit in a comfortable position on the ground or in a chair. Rest the back of your hands on your thighs. Close your eyes, if you wish.
- Gently exaggerate your next few breaths while releasing any squinting and gripping in your face, neck, and shoulders. Lengthen a few more exhales to drain your body weight down into the ground.
- Bring your awareness to your hands. Curl your fingers into gentle fists. No white knuckles. Slowly, methodically, you will unfurl one finger at a time, on one breath at a time.
- Starting with your right hand, on your next exhale, let your thumb unfurl from your palm as you mentally say, "opening." Pause in the open space at the end of your exhale. Imagine your inhalation expanding the volume of your thumb.
- On your next exhale, uncoil the right index finger, silently chanting, "opening." Relax in the pause at the end of your breath. Imagine your inhalation expanding the inner shape of your index finger.
- Continue with the next three fingers on your right hand. When your right fist has opened completely, sense the space inside your whole hand. Soft, clear, open.

- Keep your right hand open while you bring your awareness to your left hand.
- On your next exhalation, unfold your left thumb from your palm as you mentally say, "opening." Relax in the space at the end of your exhale. Welcome the inhale as you sense the volume of your thumb.
- Continue to uncurl the next four fingers with each exhale. Allow the inhale to expand you.
- When your left fist has opened completely, feel the space inside your whole hand. Soft, clear, open.
- Bring both hands into your awareness. Feel the air around your hands. Feel where your skin meets the air. Imagine that your hands are porous and you can breathe through the skin of your palms.
- For several breaths, imagine your breath flowing in through your palms up to your heart, and then from your heart back out through your hands. Imagine this path from your hands to your heart is clear, open, spacious. Unobstructed.

Pause in the open moment, at the end of the breath.
Open hands. Open mind. Open moment.

- To close, bring one hand to your heart and one to your belly. Feel your breath with your soft hands. Feel the space under your hands. Consider that you can slowly, freshly, reenter the space around you. Know that you can choose how to reenter your next moment. You can *choose* your next response.

YOGA EXPERIENCE: CHILD'S POSE

OPTIONAL PROPS: Two blankets and a block.

Sometimes, in order to open up, we actually need a moment to pull back inward. To calm, insulate, and rest. Child's pose provides a quiet moment to release effort and work, agendas and expectations and "shoulds."

- Begin on all fours. You may want to place a blanket under your knees and shins for comfort. Bring your knees together as comfortably as possible.
- Sit back on your heels and fold forward; rest your belly on your thighs completely. You may want a folded blanket (or pillow) to fill in the space between your thighs and belly.
- Place your forehead on a block on the floor and release the full weight of your head into the support. Allow your body to be held up by the ground.
- Relax here for 5 to 10 breaths and let your breath stretch the skin on your back.
- To come out of the pose, bring your hands under your shoulders, gather your belly, and slowly press up to all fours.
- Come to a seated position and bring one hand on your belly and one hand on your heart. Feel your breath in your hands. Remind yourself to stay connected to yourself as you move back into the space around you.

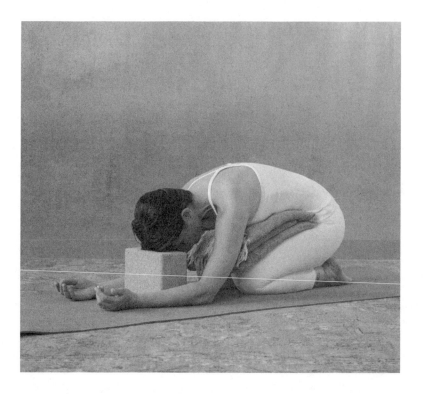

RESTORATIVE YOGA EXPERIENCE:
PROGRESSIVE RELAXATION

Progressively squeezing and releasing our major muscle groups can help us find and relieve the habitual tension that builds up throughout the day. Done often, this simple practice can uncover the deeper, historic tension we may have been carrying for years. As we regularly pause to slow down and unwind, even for a few minutes, we can create more and more space for change.

This is a short but potent practice for on-the-spot relaxation. You can do it sitting or lying down, with your eyes open or closed. It can be as short as 2 minutes, or practice as long as you would like.

- Pause and feel your body making contact with support.
- Take a few deep breaths in through your nose and out your mouth. With each exhale, you may choose to whisper the sound *ahhhh*. A soft, audible *ahhhh* can be very soothing for the nervous system and reduce overall mental and bodily tension.
- On the next three breaths, squeeze the tension out of the upper body:
- Gently make a fist on your inhale, then tense all the muscles from your knuckles to your shoulders. Shrug your shoulders up.
- On your exhale, let go completely from your shoulders to your fingers.
- Repeat three times.
- Rest for a few moments and let your breath be full and deep.
- On the next three breaths, squeeze tension out of the lower body:

- Slowly firm up your seat.
- Firm up your thighs.
- Point your toes.
- On your exhale, let your seat, thighs, and feet relax completely.
- Repeat three times.
- Rest for a few moments and let your breath be full and deep.
- Repeat these steps above, as many times as you need. If you have time, rest in full relaxation for the next several minutes.
- When you are ready to close, slowly come to a comfortable seated position. Set an intention to stay aware of your body and your breath as you transition into your day.

Journaling Prompts:
Love Your Future You

Picture a future you. Imagine that you have *already* grown in ways that allow you to feel more grounded and open, connected and whole. Imagine this more evolved you a year from now, or 5 years from now, or 10 years from now. Or more.

Pause and imagine what this future you looks like. What is your attitude and energy like?

Now write a thank-you note to your present self from Future You expressing gratitude for whatever it is that you are doing now that's laying the groundwork for your own growth and well-being. What would Future You thank Present You for?

Don't overthink it, just put your pen to paper and see what Future You has to say.

What else does your future self want you to know?

What does Future You wish for you, today, right now?

What does Future You want you to remember about your well-being?

What does Future You want you to remember about love?

Instant Pause and Reset: Come Back Here, Again

Pause to instantly reset your attention several times a day. Tracing the duration of three breaths with precision can help draw you back into the present moment, creating clarity so you can pause and *start again*.

- You can do this sitting or standing anywhere, anytime. Do a quick scan to release any obvious squinting or gripping in your face, neck, and shoulders. Let yourself land completely.
- Bring your attention to your breath and trace the length of your inhale as you mentally label its duration in three parts, "one, two, three." Notice the moment your body is fully inflated.
- As your breath shifts, trace the duration of your exhale while you mentally note, "one, two, three."
- Notice the pause at the end of your out breath. Rest in this pause until the inhale comes back to you.
- Label the duration of three full inhales and exhales.
- Pause and feel your feet on the ground as you slowly bring your awareness back into the space around you. Know that in this new, open moment, you can choose how you want to re-enter your next activity.

CHAPTER TEN

A Deep Listening Practice: Putting It All Together

Have enough courage to trust love one more time

and always one more time.

—MAYA ANGELOU

Well-being is the ability to feel okay no matter what our circumstances. To respond to the people and events in our lives from a place that's calm, clear, and open rather than react from old habits or stories that may not serve us.

The more relaxed we are, the better able we are to nurture our own well-being. True relaxation is a conscious and intentional activity. We're working with a system that is designed to not let its guard down easily.

- We begin by pausing to *welcome ourselves*, in whatever state we're in. When we feel welcomed, we show up more.
- We pause to feel our *feet on the ground—to land*—which allows us to feel safe, stable, and grounded.
- We pause to *notice our breath*, which anchors our mind in the *present moment*.

- We pause to *notice our thoughts, feelings, and any physical tension.* We remind ourselves that we don't need to fix anything, we just need to observe what arises and give it all a little more space with our breath. We practice allowing ourselves to "feel" what we feel without adding on criticism, judgment, or regret. We practice noticing how our thoughts and feelings naturally come and go when we *don't add on.*

- We practice making the choice, again and again, to go through all the steps we need to in order to *make space* for the next thing that comes up, and the next thing and the next thing.

- We practice regarding ourselves and our circumstances with *an attitude of kindness and curiosity.* We grow present and listen softly, with our eyes, ears, and heart.

- We relax our "shoulds" and our "supposed tos" and allow ourselves to *listen to what our wise, inner guidance has to say.*

- We practice regarding the people in our lives with an *attitude of compassion*—at first quietly and privately on our mat— whether we think they deserve our compassion or not. We offer compassion to the people closest to us and the people who challenge us. And we offer compassion to ourselves.

- We practice meeting our feelings, our challenges, our ideal and not-so-ideal circumstances with the intention of staying relaxed, curious, and open in the face of all of it.

- And when we're done doing all that, we get up the next day and *do it again.*

THE FULL DEEP LISTENING YOGA SEQUENCE

Done as a whole, the Deep Listening Yoga Sequence will help you cultivate a balance between stability and fluidity, strength and surrender.

It can be done at any time of the day. You can do as much or as little as your schedule and energy permit.

Listen to your breath and your body to help you make choices about which poses you may want to include or skip. And feel free to reorder the poses if you feel it is better for you.

Move slowly, so that you can *feel* what you are doing, *as* you are doing it. You can rest between poses, if you wish. Or you can move fluidly from one pose to another. Take time to pause and choose your transitions in and out of the poses, in a way that is most comfortable and natural for you.

Take your time. Quality is more healing than quantity. Remember that a little + often = a lot.

Self-care is never a selfish act—it is
simply good stewardship of the only gift
I have, the gift I was put on earth to
offer others. . . . we do it not only for
ourselves, but for the many others whose
lives we touch.

—PARKER J. PALMER

SHORT CONSTRUCTIVE REST

- Lie on your back, knees bent and leaning against each other, arms alongside your body.
- Progressively release all your body weight into the ground.
- Scan through your body for tension. Release any obvious squinting and clinching. Stay for 1 to 5 minutes.

Let the ground hold you fully.
Let your breath arrive in your body.

- Bring your hands to your belly and feel your palms receiving your breath. Imagine the breath unraveling any knots inside.
- To close, bring your knees to your belly, hugging your shins.

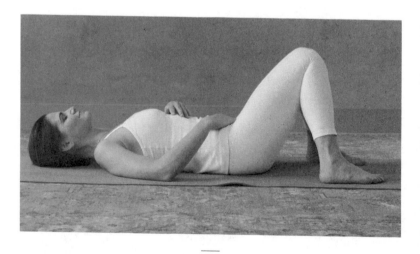

Reclining Psoas Release

- Begin in Constructive Rest.
- Bring your right knee toward your belly and interlace your hands around the back of your thigh. Your knee is bent at a 90-degree angle.
- Leave your left leg as is or, if you have no lower-back issues, extend your left leg out long, reaching actively through the heel of your left foot.
- Enjoy 5 to 10 breaths while you steadily press your right thigh into your hands.
- Then interlace your hands around your shin and hug your thigh toward your belly for another 5 to 10 breaths.
- Slowly switch to do the other side.

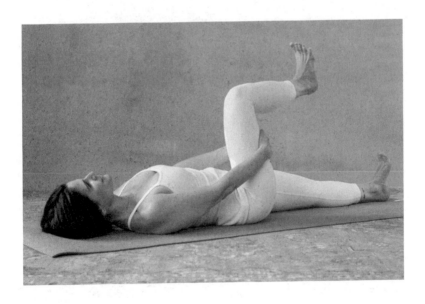

RECLINED PIGEON

- To begin, come onto your back with your knees bent, feet on the floor about hip-distance apart.
- Cross your left ankle over your right thigh. (Ensure that your left anklebone clears your right thigh completely.)
- Bring your left knee in line with your right.
- Actively flex both feet, spreading your toes and drawing them back toward your shins.
- Maintain this alignment throughout the duration of the pose.
- Stay in this shape for 5 to 10 breaths.
- Slowly transition to do the other side.

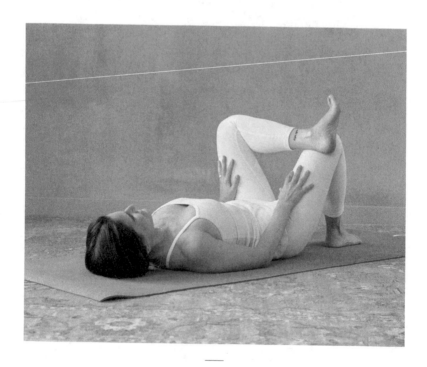

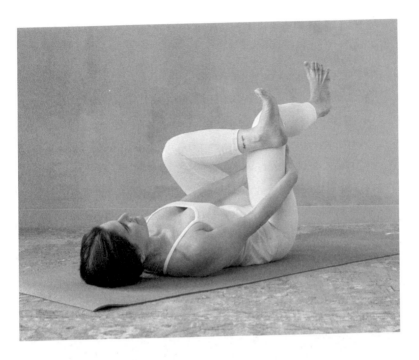

For a deeper stretch:

- Begin with the steps above, then draw your right knee toward your chest and interlace your hands behind your right hamstring.
- Gently draw your thigh toward you, maintaining your alignment from above. Allow your neck and shoulders to be at ease.
- Stay in the stretch for 5 to 10 breaths as you breathe into the sensations in your outer hip and thigh area.
- Slowly transition to do the other side.

HERO POSE

- Rest your seat on your stacked blocks.
- Draw the muscular part of your back thighs, out to the sides.
- Gently lengthen your breath as you release any tension you are holding from your head to your shoulders, shoulders to belly, and belly to seat and legs.
- Let your body rest on the ground.
- When you feel grounded, place your hands on your belly; welcome your breath.
- Relax any gripping you find in your belly. Effortless belly.

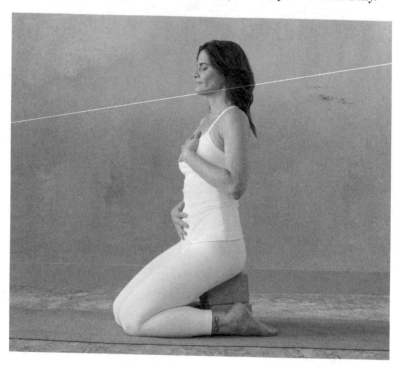

CAT/COW FLOW

- Move mindfully on your breath between Cat and Cow for a minute. Liquid, graceful, seamless.
- As you inhale, flow into cow.

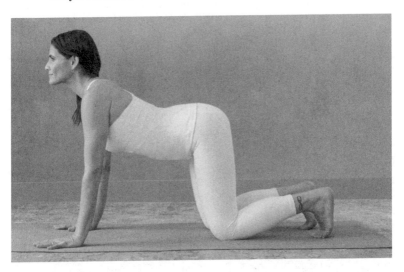

- As you exhale, flow into cat.

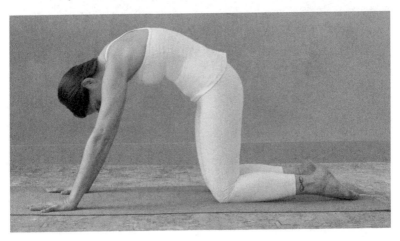

MINDFUL MOUNTAIN PAUSE

- Come to Mountain pose, and bring one hand to your belly and one hand to your chest. Feel your breath moving in and out of your hands. Welcome your breath into your hands. Enjoy 3 to 10 breaths here.

  This pause helps you stay more present in your transitions. You can use it as often as you'd like throughout your practice.

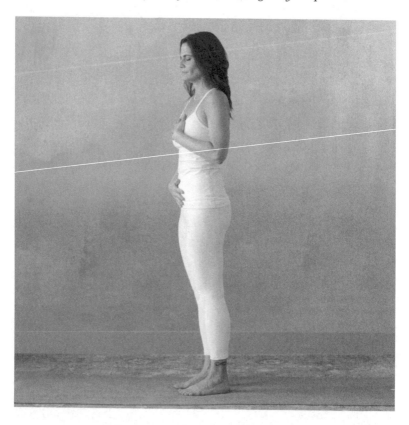

MOUNTAIN CHAIR FLOW

- Come to Mountain pose, and on your inhale lower your seat into an imaginary chair, as you sweep your arms up to the sky.
- On your exhale, rise back up to Mountain pose while sweeping your arms back down to your sides.
- Enjoy 5 to 10 breaths, flowing between Mountain and Chair.
- To finish, return to Mountain and pause.

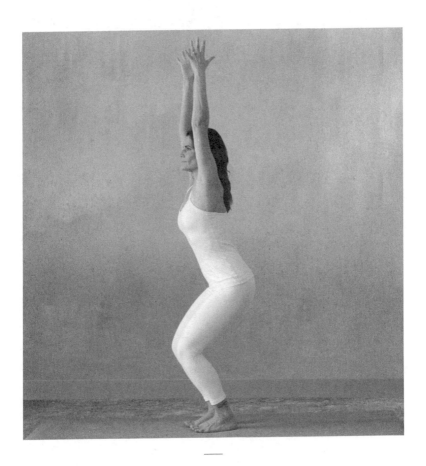

STANDING FLOWING TWIST

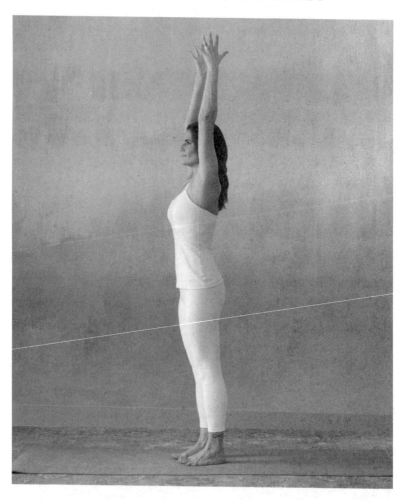

- Begin in Mountain pose.
- On your inhale, sweep your arms up; palms meet above your head.

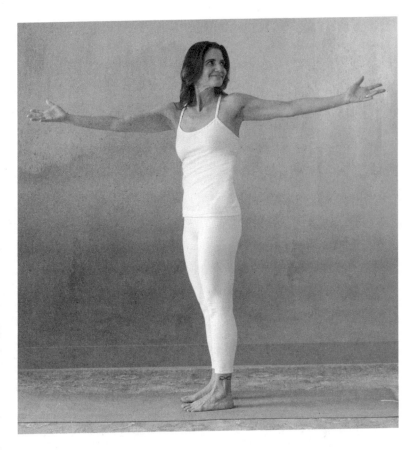

- On your exhale, twist to the right. Stretch your arms away from each other.
- Inhale sweep back up as you come center. Exhale to twist to the other side.
  - Your inhale lifts you taller, creating space for the breath.
  - Your exhale makes you wider, reaching into your twist.
- After 5 to 10 breaths of twisting, pause. Come back to Mountain.

STANDING CHEST OPENER WITH STRAP

PROP: A strap or scarf.

- Come to Mountain pose.
- Hold your strap in one hand. Bring both of your hands behind your lower back and take hold of strap with the other hand as well. Hands about shoulder-distance apart, or wider, if you need.
- From your upper arm muscles, gently and steadily pull on your strap as if you are trying to lengthen it. (Keep your grip relaxed; no white knuckles.)
  - Release any effort or tension in your neck.
  - Collarbones widen toward your shoulders.
  - Visualize three long breaths moving through imaginary nostrils on your chest center.
- Slowly release the strap from one hand.
- Pause in Mountain and enjoy a few breaths. Allow your strong legs to carry your light and open shoulders and chest.

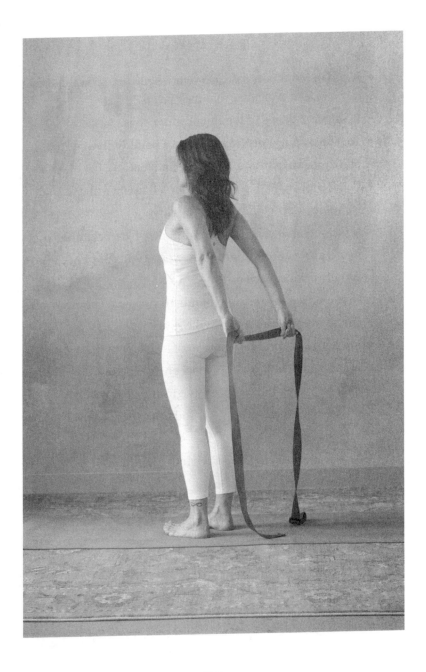

TREE POSE

- Begin in Mountain pose. Let your weight drain down into your legs and feet, expanding into their prints.
- Bring your hands to the rim of your pelvis.
- To help balance, rest your eyes on a point in front of you.
- Shift your weight to your left leg and foot.
- Bring your right heel up onto your left ankle while the ball of right foot stays connected to the floor.
- If you feel stable, bring the entire sole of your right foot onto your calf or inner thigh. Press your right foot and left leg equally against each other.
- If you'd like, bring your hands to prayer position at your chest or reach your arms to the sky.
- For up to 10 breaths, notice what happens in your body, mind, and breath when you feel unsteady. How do you "hold on"? Simply notice, without judgment, what you are "adding on" to this situation, let it be, and bring yourself back to your breath.
- To release the pose, step back into Mountain. Repeat on the opposite side.

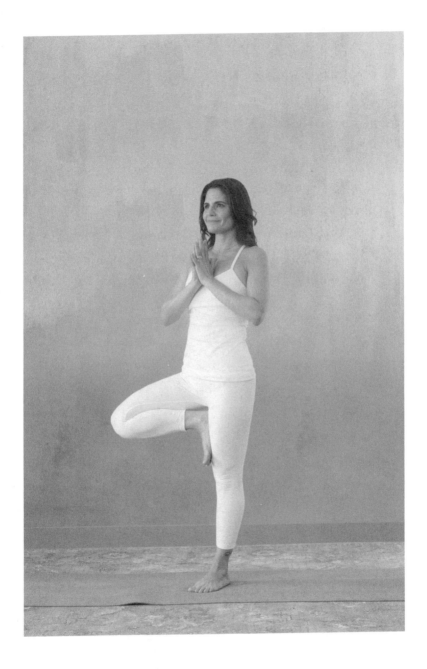

FLOWING WARRIOR 2

- Begin in Warrior 2.

Firm the backs of your thighs and your seat. Let your strong legs hold your light upper body.

LET'S FLOW

- On your inhalation, push the ground down to straighten your legs and sweep your arms up to the sky.
- On your exhale, return to Warrior 2.
- Continue to flow in and out of Warrior 2, synchronizing your movement with your breath. Repeat 5 to 10 times.

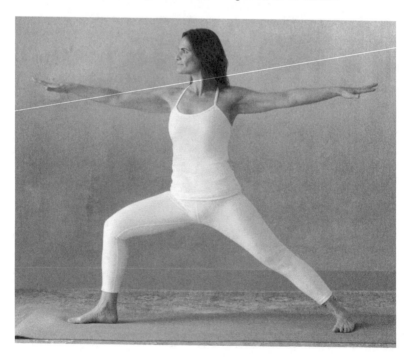

- Pause in Warrior 2 for a few last breaths. Ask yourself: Where can I be more stable? Where can I be more open?
- Slowly transition to do the other side.

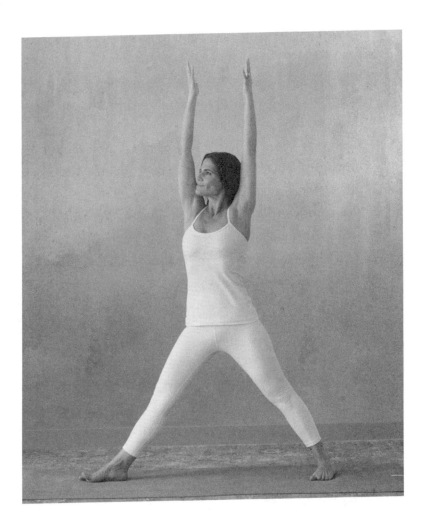

Standing Wide-Leg Forward Bend

PROPS: Two blocks

- Come to Mountain pose, facing the long edge of your mat.
- Place your blocks, in their highest height, a few inches in front of your feet.
- Extend your arms out to the sides of your body in a T shape.
- Step your legs wide apart, bringing your ankles directly under your wrists with the outer edges of your feet parallel to the short edges of your mat.
- Bend your knees deeply and fold forward from your hips, bringing your hands to the blocks. Slide your blocks directly under your shoulders.
- Keep your pelvis in line with your heels as you extend your spine long, parallel to the ground like a tabletop. You may keep your knees bent. Or you may straighten your legs, as long as that doesn't round your back.
  - Firm the muscles of the bottom half of your seat and the back of your upper thighs.
  - Spread into your footprints.
  - Elongate from your tail to your crown.
- Lengthen your breath on purpose so you feel the skin on your back stretched by your breath. Stay here for 5 to 10 breaths.
- When you are ready to come out, bend your knees, bring your hands to your thighs, and slowly come back up to a tall posture.
- Step your feet together. Pause in Mountain.

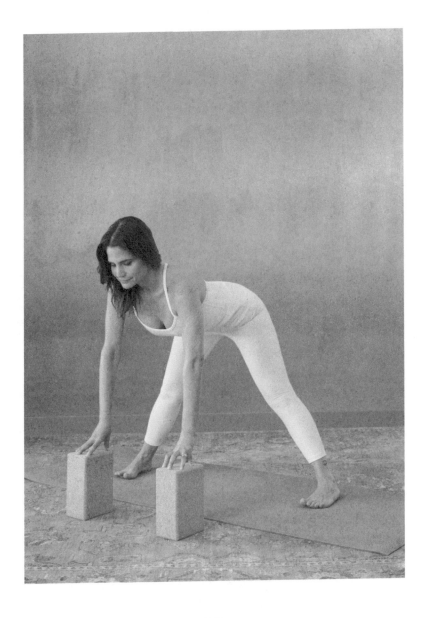

DOWN DOG

- Come to all fours, hands a little wider than your shoulders, knees about as wide as your hips. Curl the balls of your feet into the ground.
- Push down into your hands and feet as you gather your belly, up into your pelvis, drawing your hips up to the sky.
- You are now in an upside-down V shape. Bend your knees, if that's more comfortable.
- Spread your toes and actively explore how it feels to lift your heels high, coming up onto the balls of the feet.
- Lengthen from your legs from your pelvis through the balls of your feet, into the ground.
- Reach from your heart through your hands, down into the earth.
- Enjoy 5 to 10 breaths here.
- Before you lower, gather your belly again, then slowly come back to all fours and transition to the next pose.

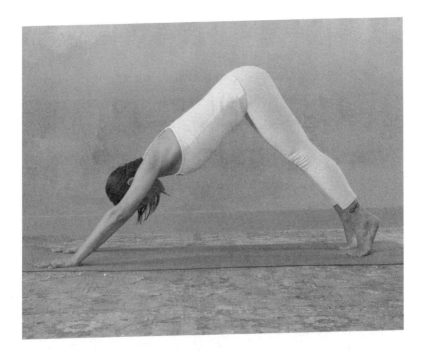

LOW LUNGE

- Begin on all fours. Step your left foot between your hands. Bring your hands to the blocks.
- Your front knee lines up over your ankle.
- Press the ball of your back foot into your mat.
- *Firm* the bottom of your seat and back upper thighs.
  - Let your weight drain down.
  - Your upper body is light.
- After 5 to 10 breaths, come back to all fours. Repeat on the other side.

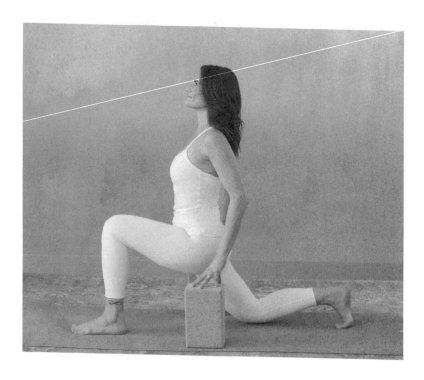

GECKO ARM FLOWING COBRA

- Lie on your belly. Stretch your legs long, hands in line with your breastbone. Come onto your fingertips.
- On each inhale, press your pelvis, legs, and fingertips down as your chest floats up.
- There's no need to overeffort or pull yourself up. Like a balloon, your breath will float you up.
- On each exhalation, lengthen your lower back as you lower down.
- Repeat 5 to 10 times.

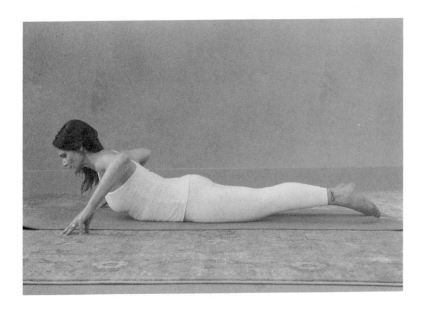

CHILD'S POSE

OPTIONAL PROPS: Two blankets (or pillows) and a block.

- Come to all fours.
- Sit back on your heels and fold forward; rest your belly on your thighs. You may want a folded blanket (or pillow) to fill in the space between your thighs and belly.
- Place your forehead on a block or the floor and release the full weight of your head into the support. Relax and let your breath stretch the skin on your back.
- Allow your body to be held up by the ground.
- Relax here for 5 to 10 breaths.

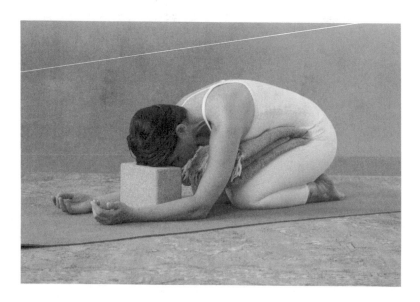

RESTORATIVE:
FULL-BODY RELAXATION

- To begin, set up two blocks side by side at the foot of your mat and place your short-roll blanket on top of them. Slowly lower yourself to the floor. Mindfully take your legs over the roll. Place a pillow under your head and neck, if you like.
- Rest your arms by your sides, or place your hands on your belly, with elbows on the floor.
- Make adjustments to ensure you are comfortable. Take several long breaths as you progressively release all of your body weight onto the ground.
- *Relax more* for the next 5 to 20 minutes.

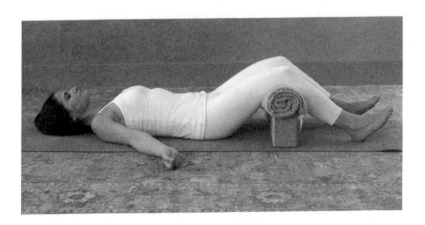

Relaxmore
Expand Into Yourself and Relax More

Let your body land on the ground.

Allow your heels to be *held completely*.
Your legs and pelvis
dropping into the ground.

Your back
spreading across the floor.
The ground will hold you up.

Let your upper back,
shoulders,
and head
rest completely
on the ground.

The ground longs to carry you,
so your breath can fill you.

Welcome your breath into your body.
Let the waves of breath
flow freely on their own.

Nothing to resist.
Nothing to do.

Feel where your skin meets the air.
Imagine you could breathe through your skin.

———

Porous skin.

Porous body.

Porous mind.

Porous heart.

Soften into the wholeness

that you are.

Expanding

into

yourself.

You are bigger than you think you are.

You are already whole.

You are already whole.

A SUPPLE PSOAS SEQUENCE

If you are looking for a shorter practice or need a more calming practice, try this sequence, which focuses on releasing excess tension in the psoas muscles and gently opening your body for full, complete breathing.

- Short Constructive Rest
- Reclining Psoas Release
- Reclined Pigeon
- Hero
- Cat/Cow Flow
- Mindful Mountain Pause
- Standing Flowing Twist
- Low Lunge

RESTORATIVE:
FINISH WITH ALL OR ANY OF THESE POSES.

- Restorative: Constructive Rest (5 to 10 minutes)
- Restorative: Surfboard (5 to 10 minutes)
- Restorative: Legs up on a Chair (5 to 10 minutes)

HOW TO PREPARE FOR
YOUR PRACTICE

TAKE TIME FOR YOU

The best time to practice is anytime you can commit to it regularly. Personally, I like to practice first thing in the morning, as it sets the tone for my day and ensures that I don't get sidetracked by responsibilities and distractions.

What is important is regularity. Find a 10- to 30-minute slot in your day that you can dedicate to your practice. If you can stretch out one to three longer practices (20 to 60 minutes) during the week, add those in to your weekly schedule. Remember, a little + often = a lot.

CREATING YOUR SPACE

The more comfortable and happy you are in your practice space, the more you will want to show up there. Think of this as a special space where you feel cared for and at ease. Choose a spot that is private, warm, and quiet. It's helpful if there are no phones or distracting devices. You should have enough space to stand on your yoga mat and reach in all directions.

It's lovely to add some personal heart-warming objects to your space, such as photos of loved ones, a special rock from a hike, maybe flowers. I recommend keeping a journal near your mat. I find that after practice my mind and heart are open, and writing comes more easily. Sometimes I get a flow of insight as I am practicing, and I pause to make a note in my journal while these thoughts are fresh.

Props

You can find yoga props online, at your local yoga studio, or at a sporting goods store. However, you can also use items from around the house.

YOGA MAT: I recommend practicing on an actual yoga mat, as their grip offers more safety than a towel or carpet.

YOGA STRAP: For this practice, you don't need a fancy strap. You can buy one if you wish, but truly, a belt or scarf will do.

YOGA BLOCKS: Yoga blocks are made from wood, cork, or foam. I find that foam is most comfortable for use underneath the body in resting poses.

YOGA BLANKETS: Yoga blankets and traditional Mexican blankets are made of finely woven wool or cotton and offer consistent, even support. However, you can use oversize beach towels as well, if they have a consistent, even density.

Bed pillows are great replacements for blankets in many poses, too. Usually, a king- or queen- size pillow will work best. However, ensure that the pillow offers consistent support and that its fill is not lumpy or uneven.

BLANKET FOLDING

Long Rectangle—Folded Blanket

- Open your yoga blanket fully.
- Fold the blanket in half widthwise, bringing the fringed sides together. Line up the blanket corners precisely. Turn the blanket so that the fringe hangs toward the floor.
- Fold the blanket in half lengthwise, with the fringe continuing to hang toward the floor.
- Fold the blanket in half lengthwise again, the fringe still toward the floor.

Short Rectangle—Folded Blanket

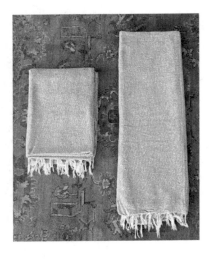

- Fold the blanket according to the long rectangle instructions, above.
- Then fold the blanket in half, down toward the fringe. The fringe still hangs toward the floor as you create a shorter rectangle.

Long-Roll Blanket

- Open your yoga blanket fully.
- Fold the blanket in half widthwise, bringing the fringed sides together. Line up the blanket corners precisely. Turn the blanket so that the fringe hangs toward the floor.
- Roll the blanket lengthwise, so that the fringe is at one short end of the roll.

Short-Roll Blanket

- Open your yoga blanket fully.
- Fold the blanket in half widthwise, bringing the fringed sides together. Line up the corners precisely. Turn the blanket so that the fringe hangs toward the floor.

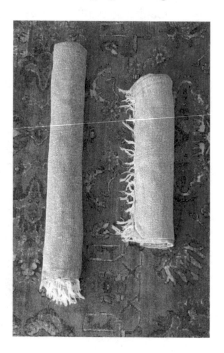

- Fold the blanket in half lengthwise, with the fringe continuing to hang toward the floor.
- Roll it like a yoga mat, toward the fringe.
- Your short roll will have fringe along the full length of the roll.

Setting Up Your Meditation Seat

Personally, I meditate everywhere, which means I sit on everything from chairs and train seats to meditation cushions and blankets. If you choose a chair, it is ideal if your feet can rest completely on the ground (or on blocks) and that you have good back support. You should feel comfortable and at ease. My favorite go-to meditation setup is to sit against the wall, adding support under my seat, knees, and arms. Here's how:

- Stack three folded blankets and place them against a wall.
- Sit cross-legged with one block under each knee for support.
- Place blocks or pillows on top of your thighs to rest your forearms on. This will take strain off the shoulders and neck.

For recordings of the meditations I share in the book, please visit jillianpransky.com/deeplisteningmeditations.

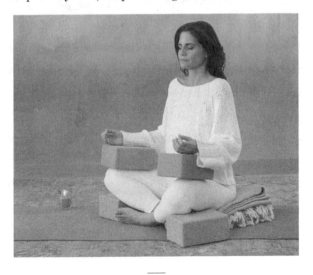

ACKNOWLEDGMENTS

Thank *you* for meeting me here and embarking on this healing practice. There are many people who have made it possible for me to share this work with you for whom I have deep gratitude.

I AM FOREVER GRATEFUL TO MY TEACHERS

I have been blessed with the opportunity to study with some the greatest yoga and meditation masters of our time, all of whom I have deep gratitude for. And while they have each contributed to my growth, I would like to pay tribute to those who have made profound, lasting impacts on my personal practice and what I share as a teacher to date.

I am grateful to my first meditation lineage and practice, Transcendental Meditation, and the mantra I received at 9 years old (which I still call upon today when I need extra support focusing or calming anxiety).

I was gifted to begin my path with Yogi Raj Alan Finger. His integration of yoga, meditation, and Ayurveda is a foundation of my approach to yoga as a healing art. I will be forever grateful for the Yoga Zone community and all the teachers and students who I 'grew up' with.

From my very first class with the luminous Erich Schiffmann in 1996, I was home. Erich's *Moving into Stillness* was a pinnacle shift for me. Erich introduced me to yoga as a path of receptivity, attunement, and love, rather than executing, accomplishing, and qualifying.

Also in 1996, I began a decade of work with the brilliant Dr. Ruella Frank, founder of the Center for Somatic Studies. Through my work with Ruella, I gained a deep understanding of the connection between our emotions and behaviors to our movement patterns and somatic experience. I learned to stay present with and digest the difficult emotions and sensations that often come up on the mat and cushion. Ruella has taught me magnitudes about forgiveness of both myself and others, and how to care for the parts of myself that I had habitually rejected. In short, she was a master at holding the space for me to listen deeply and bravely, again and again.

In my 20s, an incredible wave of opportunities to study with several luminaries continued to come my way. I am particularly grateful to the teachings of Jon Kabat-Zinn, Jack Kornfield, Ram Dass, and especially Sharon Salzberg. It was after my first 5-day silent retreat with Sharon that I grew more committed to Buddhist meditation. Her philosophies of kindness, self-acceptance, and presence continue to inspire me daily. My practice and teaching today is also greatly influenced by the beautiful work of Tara Brach.

My practice of Deep Listening truly evolved when I began to integrate the work of Pema Chödrön. In 1998, Omega Institute invited me to lead the yoga program during Pema's retreat. In order to craft yoga classes that would enrich her students' experience, I read her book *When Things Fall Apart*. She had me at page one. The opportunity to receive her teachings and immediately incorporate them into my yoga classes exponentially elevated my absorption of her work. After that weekend with her, I knew I had found my teacher. But what I didn't know then was that I'd be invited to lead the yoga classes during her program annually for the next 20 years. I am forever humbled and inspired by her humanity, mastery, generosity, and compassion.

As a yoga therapist and teacher trainer, I study the work of healers, doctors, and neurologists in order to draw from the most up-to date research in mind-body medicine. I am particularly thankful for the work of Doctors Herbert Benson, Daniel Siegel, Richard Davidson, and Rick Hanson.

My students, especially those who have shared this path with me for decades, are a constant source of insight, inspiration, and friendship for me. I send a loving thank you to my retreat communities— Race Brook, Isla Mujeres, Tulum, Costa Rica, Blue Spirit, Kripalu, Omega, Mohonk Mountain House, as well as all my students from almost 25 years of classes and trainings, most notably at Hoboken YMCA, Yoga Zone, Devotion Yoga, Be Yoga, YogaWorks, JaiPure Yoga, Kaia Yoga, Elevate Yoga, and Dig Yoga.

A huge heartfelt thank you all the Bright Spirits from the Hoboken Y and Devotion Yoga. To Liza Bertini. And most especially to my dear friends Carrie Parker Gastelu, my collaborator and partner, and Tam Terry, a profound teacher of generosity and dedication.

I Am Grateful to Those Who Help Bring My Work to Others

There have been so many people behind the scenes supporting me, managing my events, promoting my programs, and making sure my work gets out in to the world. Some of these folks have been with me for many years—I offer a very special thank you to Rasmani Debbie Orth and Luke Breslin at Kripalu, Jessica Smith and Julie Wood at YogaWorks, and Brett Bevell at Omega.

Also behind the curtains has been Maya Magennis, Erin Polychronopoulos, Christine Engelfried, Jill Bauman, and Veronica Perretti. As well as Lourdes Soares, Julie Delaney Baccaglini, and Jessica Dixion Majka.

A Huge bow is extended to all the amazing teachers who volunteer to assist my programs, workshops, trainings, and retreats. Each of you has contributed to my growth as a teacher and enabled me to offer more of myself to others. Thank you.

And a special thank you to a few others who have truly supported my programs and work: Scott Chesney, Maureen Primrose, Jenny Pop, and Lisa Weinert.

I Am Grateful to Those Who Helped Me Bring This Book into Being

When I first received my offer to write *Deep Listening* with Rodale, I knew that I needed Jessica Wolf on board to help me. Her friendship, expertise, wisdom, and masterful writing have been essential in bringing this book to life. For over 20 years, my path has been unusually blessed by the mentorship, support, and love of Jessica, and of the whole Wolf Webb Family.

Thank you to my agent Maria Ribas at Stonesong for believing in my concept and helping to find the right publisher. Thank you to

Rodale Books and Leah Miller for wanting to share my voice and teaching with the world. And most especially, thank you to my editor Anna Cooperberg. Anna's clarity, passion and love for yoga was just what *Deep Listening* needed to come into full bloom. More gratitude to publisher Gail Gonzales, editorial director Jennifer Levesque, and the rest of the fantastic team at Rodale: Amy King, Carol Angstadt, Marilyn Hauptly, Angie Giammarino, Brianne Sperber, and Emily Eagan.

Huge thank you to my friends at MacMillan for helping to bring my book to the shelves. At the time of signing with Rodale, I didn't realize that my old friends and co-workers from St. Martin's Press would wind up being a most essential conduit for my work to spread in the world (Matthew Shear would have gotten a kick out that!).

Both Jessica and I are grateful to the many friends who helped refine this work. Huge thank you to Nancy Friedman, Jodi Bienenfield, and the Tuesday Night Writing Group including Pam, Kathleen, Jennifer, Valerie, Linda, and Laura.

The Heart of My Teaching

My personal relationships have been the most significant catalyst for bringing my yoga to life. I am grateful to all of my family and dear friends who have helped me grow as a person and who have shared this path with me.

Most importantly, my very first teachers: my parents, Paul and Phyllis, and my brothers, Scott and Bennett. And my extended family:

Scott & Danielle and Bennett, Kelly & Easton. Bob & Anne, Norma, and Jodi, Zach & Josh. I offer a special embrace to Nicole Alley Farrah, Jodi Bienenfield, and the whole Highmont Terrace Gang.

Lastly, with a huge heart, I extend my love and gratitude to my husband Brad, my son William, and our cuddly pup Sunday.

I am grateful for the blessing of my son William. He is a brilliant, bold, creative force of life that may shape me perhaps more than I shape him. He continues to expand my capacity to pause, be humble, and lead with love.

I am thankful to Brad, my sweetheart, who has witnessed, challenged, coached, cheerleaded, and celebrated my evolution for 25 years. Our marriage and experience as parents has given me the great opportunity to practice every skill I have ever learned on the mat and cushion. I am forever grateful for his love, friendship, humor, support, steadfastness, and wisdom. Brad is also the one who literally put this book in motion—he threw me out of the nest and on to the path to publish *Deep Listening*.

INDEX

Boldface page references denote photographs.

A

Adrenaline, 30
Adversity, metaphor for meeting, 132
Alertness, holding ourselves in, 79
Anxiety
    addressing by focusing on our body,
        57–58
    breathing and, 50–51, 57–58
Anxiety attack, 10–12
Asthma, 51
Attention
    Chinese sign for, 131
    Creating Space Meditation Experience,
        117–18
    listening with our heart, 131
    loving, 150
    to our breath, 52, 57–60
    pausing to reset, 101
    space between the notes, 156
Awareness, 224–25

B

Back pain, from tight psoas, 35
Barenblat, Rachel, 189
Barriers, removing, 185–87
Being here, 49–74
    bringing your mind home with
        breathing, 52
    message, 62–63
    paying attention to our breath, 52,
        57–60
    practices for, 64–74
        Contemplation, 64
        Instant Pause and Reset, 74
        Journaling Prompt, 73
        Meditation Experience, 66–67
        Relaxmore, 72–73
    Restorative Yoga Experience, 70,
        70–71
    Yoga Experience, 68–69, 68–69
    reasons for failure to stay here, 55–56
    returning to here, 61
Belly breathing, soft, 167–68
Blankets, yoga, 8–9, 264–66, 265–66
Blocks, yoga, 8, 264, 267, 267
Blood draw, author's experience with,
        75–76, 80–82, 84, 86
Body awareness, 224–25
Brach, Tara, 28, 132, 269
Brain, as thought factory, 81–82
Breathing
    anxiety and, 50–51, 57–58
    Being with the Flow of Your Breath,
        66–67
    bringing your mind home with, 52
    connectedness and, 59
    ever-constant, ever-changing nature
        of, 60
    heart breathing, 151
    Listening to Your Breath, 62–63
    making room for breath to expand in
        heart center, 146–47
    mindful, 57–58
    paying attention to our breath, 52,
        57–60
    as process we allow to happen, 59–60
    to reset your attention and presence, 74
    returning to here, 61
    soft belly, 167–68
    synchronizing our movement with
        breath, 144–45

C

Calmness, 36
Cat/Cow Flow, 68–69, 68–69, 241, 241

Change, 55–56, 216
Chest-opening pose, Easy Fish Pose as, 146–47, **147**
Child's Pose, 226, **227**, 258, **258**
Clarity, 36
Clinging, 112–13
Clothes, too-tight, 78–81, 86
Compassion, 180–82, 190, 209, 233
    choosing, 189
    Journaling Prompt, 206
    metta meditation, 183–84
Compassion practice, 190
Connectedness
    awareness of breathing and, 59
    experiencing, 2
    metta meditation, 183
Constructive Rest, 22–23, **23**, 236, **236**
Contemplations
    being here, 64
    description of, 7
    landing on the ground, 38
    listening again and again and again, 222–23
    listening bravely, 194–95
    listening deeply, 166
    listening softly, 140–41
    making space, 116
    noticing how we hold, 90
    in sample weekly practice schedule, 9
    welcoming ourselves, 17
Contentment, 13–14
Control
    feeling out of control, 110–11
    illusion of, 55
    wired for, 113
Cortisol, 30
Creativity, 214
Curiosity, 133–34, 136, 157–58, 166, 233

D

Deep Listening Yoga Sequence, 234–58
    Cat/Cow Flow, 241, **241**
    Child's Pose, 258, **258**
    Constructive Rest, 236, **236**
    Down Dog, 254, **255**
    Flowing Warrior 2, 250–51, **250-51**
    Gecko Arm Flowing Cobra, 257, **257**
    Hero Pose, 240, **240**
    Low Lunge, 256, **256**

Mindful Mountain Pause, 242, **242**
Mountain Chair Flow, 243, **243**
Reclined Pigeon, 238–39, **238-39**
Reclining Psoas Release, 237, b237
Standing Chest Opener with Strap, 246–47, **247**
Standing Flowing Twist, 244–45, **244-45**
Standing Wide-Leg Forward Bend, 252, **253**
Tree Pose, 248, **248**
Digestion, hampered by tight psoas, 35
Do-over, 212
Down Dog, 254, **255**

E

Easy Chest Opener, **70**, 70–71
Easy Fish Pose, 146–47, **147**
Empathy, 189
Epinephrine, 30
Equanimity, 14
Equipment, 8, 264–66
Evolving, 2, 182, 210, 212, 214, 216, 223

F

Fear, 11–12
Feeling(s), 157–61, 233
    fluidity of, 161
    mindful yoga practice and, 157
    pausing to welcome, 164
Fight, flight, or flee response, 30–31, 34
Flower, visualization of blooming, 194–95
Flowing Warrior 2, **169**, 169–72, **171**, 250–51, **250-51**
Full Relaxation, **122**, 122–23

G

Gecko Arm Flowing Cobra, 144–45, **144-45**, 257, **257**
Goddess Pose, **173**, 173–75
Ground, our relationship with the, 33
Grounding
    benefits of, 35–36
    Journaling Prompt: Finding Groundedness, 47

Grounding *(cont.)*
  Meditation Experience: Hourglass
    Meditation, 39
  paying attention to our breath, 52,
    57–60
  releasing tension, 104
Guided relaxation, 6–7

H

Happiness, 13
Heart, listening with, 131
Heart breaths, 151
Heart center, 146
Heart practice, 131
Helicopter wisdom, 154–55, 163–64, 166
Hero Pose, 20, **21**, 240, **240**
Hourglass Mediation, 39
House metaphor, 32
How We Hold, 75–101
  conversations with our thoughts, 81–86
  living in too-tight clothes, 80–81
  message, 88–89
  90-second rule, 84
  noticing where we hold, 86–87
  practices for noticing, 90–101
    Contemplation, 90
    Instant Pause and Reset, 101
    Journaling Prompts, 100
    Meditation Experience, 91–92
    Relaxmore, 98–99
    Restorative Yoga Experience, **96**,
      96–97
    Yoga Experience, 93, **94**, 95
  tension sources, 77–78

I

Inner voice, 7, 132, 153, 155, 158
Instant Pause and Reset
  Be Here Now, 74
  Come Back Here, Again, 231
  description of, 8
  Effortless Support, 48
  heart breathing, 151
  Metta Expansion, 207
  Open, Listen, Choose, 179
  Open Sky, 127

Paying Careful Attention, 101
  in sample weekly practice schedule, 9
  A Warm Greeting, 26
Intentional community, 53
Intention setting, 214–15

J

Journal, 264
Journaling Prompt
  Create Spaciousness, 126
  description of, 7
  Finding Groundedness, 47
  Growing Present, 73
  Invite Your Authentic Self, 25
  for listening bravely, 206
  Love Your Future You, 230
  Loving Attention, 150
  Meeting Your Tension, 100
  Open to Receive, 178
  in sample weekly practice schedule, 9

K

Kindness, 189, 191, 233
  benefits of attitude of, 136
  listening with, 132–33
Knots, 71, 128–30, 135, 142

L

Labeling, 91–92, 101
Landing, 37–47
  message, 37
  our relationship with the ground, 33
  practices for landing on the ground,
    38–48
    Contemplation, 38
    Instant Pause and Reset, 48
    Journaling Prompts, 47
    Meditation Experience, 39
    Relaxmore, 46
    Restorative Yoga Experience,
      44–45, **44–45**
    Yoga Experience, **40**, 41–42, **43**
Legs up on a Chair, **96**, 96–97
Lessing, Doris, 186

Letting go, making space *versus*, 108
Letting things be, 108, 110, 129
Listening
    Chinese character for, 131
    compassionate, 131, 150
    with curiosity, 133–34, 158
    kindly, 132–33, 158
    with our heart, 131
    during stillness, 129
Listening again and again and again,
    208–31
    future starts now, 216
    intention setting, 214–15
    message, 218–21
    practices for, 222–31
        Contemplation, 222–23
        Instant Pause and Rest, 231
        Journaling Prompt, 230
        Meditation Experience, 224–25
        Restorative Yoga Experience,
           228–29
        Yoga Experience, 226, **227**
Listening bravely
    compassion, 180–82, 189
    message, 192–93
    metta meditation, 183–85, 187–88,
        195–99
    practices for, 194–207
        Contemplation, 194–95
        Instant Pause and Reset, 207
        Journaling Prompt, 206
        Meditation Experience, 195–99
        Relaxmore, 204–5
        Restorative Yoga Experience,
           202–3, **203**
        Yoga Experience, 200–201, **201**
    Princess and the Dragon (fable),
        180–82
    removing our barriers, 185–87
Listening deeply, 152–71
    broadening of our perspective by,
        162–63
    feeling(s), 157–61
    helicopter wisdom, 154–55
    message, 164–65
    mindful yoga practice, 157–58
    practices for, 166–79
        Contemplation, 166
        Instant Pause and Reset, 179
        Journaling Prompts, 178

        Meditation Experience, 167–68
        Relaxmore, 176–77
        Restorative Yoga Experience, **173**,
           173–75
        Yoga Experience, **169**, 169–72,
           171
    space between the notes, 156
    static of "no," 155
    what we need to know, 161–62
Listening practice, 130, 178
Listening softly, 128–51
    developing a listening practice, 130
    listening with our heart, 131
    message, 138–39
    practices for, 140–51
        Contemplation, 140–41
        Instant Pause and Reset, 151
        Journaling Prompts, 150
        Meditation Experience, 142–43
        Relaxmore, 148–49
        Restorative Yoga Experience,
           146–47, **147**
        Yoga Experience, 144–45,
           144–45
Low Lunge, 200–201, **201**, 256, **256**

M

Making space, 102–27, 233
    letting go *versus*, 108
    meeting our stillness, 106
    message, 115
    practices for, 116–27
        Contemplation, 116
        Instant Pause and Reset Open Sky,
           127
        Journaling Prompts, 126
        Meditation Experience, 117–18
        Relaxmore, 124–25
        Restorative Yoga Experience, **122**,
           122–23
        Yoga Experience, 119, **120–21**
    reason for, 114
    releasing tension, 104
    solution for, 113
Mantra, for staying present with your
    breath, 66–67
Meditation, metta, 183–85, 187–88,
    195–99

Meditation Experience
    Being with the Flow of Your Breath,
        66–67
    Creating Space, 117–18
    description of, 6
    Elevator to a Welcoming Arrival, 17–19
    Hourglass Meditation, 39
    Listening Openly Softly, Wholly,
        142–43
    Metta, 195–99
    Noticing and Labeling, 91–92
    Open Hands, Open Mind, Open Heart,
        224–25
    in sample weekly practice schedule, 9
    Soft Belly Breathing, 167–68
Meditation seat, 267, **267**
Metta Expansion, 207
Metta meditation, 183–85, 187–88,
        195–99
Mind-body connection, 32–33
Mind-body conversation, 34–35
Mindful breathing, 57–58
Mindful Mountain Pause, 242, **242**
Mindfulness, 53–54, 131
Mindful yoga practice, 157–58
Motivation, 213
Mountain Chair Flow, 42, **43**, 243, **243**
Mountain Pose, **40**, 41
Muscle tension, 77
Muscle tightness, 77

N

Nhat Hanh, Thich, 53, 61, 216
90-second rule, 84
"No," static of, 155
Noticing
    stillness and, 132
    thoughts, 85–86, 91–92
    where we hold, 86–87, 104

P

Panic attack, 10–12, 28, 129, 135
Pausing. *See also* Instant Pause and Reset
    benefits of, 14–15
    for do-over, 212
    to notice thoughts, 85–86

to replace our attention on breathing, 52
to welcome feelings, 164
Perspective, broadening by listening
        deeply, 162–63
Practices
    for being here, 64–74
    benefits of daily, 3–4
    for landing on the ground, 38–48
    for listening bravely, 194–207
    for listening deeply, 166–79
    for listening softly, 140–51
    for making space, 116–27
    for noticing how we hold, 90–101
    overview of, 6–8
    preparing for practice, 263–67
    sample weekly practice schedule, 9
    for welcoming ourselves, 17–26
Practice space, 263–64
Princess and the Dragon (fable), 180–82
Progressive relaxation, 228–29
Props, 8, 264–66
Protection
    clinging and, 113
    making space, 104
    tension and, 77, 100, 130
    thoughts and, 83
    vulnerability and, 111
Psoas muscle, 34–35, 54, 57, 116, 122
    Reclining Psoas Release, 237, **237**
    Supple Psoas Sequence, 262

R

Reclined Pigeon, 238–39, **238–39**
Reclining Psoas Release, 237, **237**
Relaxation
    art of, 104
    as conscious and intentional activity,
        232
    feeling out of control, 110–11
    full-body, 259, **259**
    Full Relaxation Restorative Yoga
        Experience, **122**, 122–23
    grounding and, 36
    listening practice, 130
    meeting our stillness, 106
    progressive, 228–29
    Restorative Yoga Experience, 202–3,
        203

Relaxation response, 32, 114
Relaxmore
    Be Here and Relax More, 72–73
    benefits of use, 7
    Expand Into Yourself and Relax More,
        260–61
    Land and Relax More, 46
    Listen Bravely and Relax More, 204–5
    Listening Deeply and Relax More,
        176–77
    Listen Softly and Relax More, 148–49
    Make Space and Relax More, 124–25
    Notice and Relax More, 98–99
    Show Up and Relax More, 24
Release, psoas muscle, 34–35
Reset. *See* Instant Pause and Reset
Rest, constructive, 22–23, **23**, 236, **236**
Restlessness, 30
Restorative Yoga Experience
    Constructive Rest, 22–23, **23**
    description of, 6–7
    Easy Chest Opener, **70**, 70–71
    Easy Fish Pose, 146–47, **147**
    finishing poses, 262
    Full-Body Relaxation, 259, **259**
    Full Relaxation, **122**, 122–23, 202–3,
        203
    Goddess Pose, **173**, 173–75
    Legs up on a Chair, **96**, 96–97
    progressive relaxation, 228–29
    in sample weekly practice schedule, 9
    Surfboard, 44–45, **44–45**
Roth, Jeff, 189

S

Salty solution metaphor, 109
Savasana, author's first, 102–3, 106
Schiffmann, Erich, 154, 159
Schnabel, Arthur, 156–57
Self-care, 235
Setting intentions, 214–15
Soft Belly Breathing, 167–68
Softness, required for tension release, 135
Space between the notes, 156
Standing Chest Opener with Strap,
    246–47, **247**
Standing Flowing Twist, 119, **120–21**,
    244–45, **244–45**

Standing Wide-Leg Forward Bend, 252,
    253
Stillness, 106
    listening during, 129
    noticing during, 132
Strap, yoga, 9, 264
Stress
    manifestations of, 30
    psoas muscle tightening with, 57
    reacting rather than responding, 31
    response to, 2, 130, 136
        in our body, 31–32
        in our mind, 30–31
        speed of, 57
    sources of
        inner voices, 132
        restricted breathing, 51
Stress hormones, 30, 74, 78
Supple Psoas Sequence, 262
Surfboard, 44–45, **44–45**

T

Taylor, Jill Bolte, 84
Tension, 76–80
    author's experiences with, 103
    Meeting Your Tension (Journaling
        Prompt), 100
    noticing where we hold, 86–87, 104
    protection and, 77, 100, 130
    releasing, 106
        as act of consciously making space,
            104
        in back and psoas, 96–97, 122
        essential components to, 105
        by pausing, 15
        with progressive relaxation, 228–29
        results of, 114
        softness required for, 135
        vulnerability associated with, 111
    results of, 80, 103, 114
    sources of, 77–78, 106, 108, 111, 132
    tight-clothes metaphor, 78–81
    tightness compared, 77
Thoughts
    brain as thought factory, 81–82
    conversations with our, 81–86
    labeling, 91–92
    negative, 83

Thoughts *(cont.)*
90-second rule, 84
noticing, 85–86, 91–92
repeat, 82–83
Tightness, muscle, 77
Toolbox, Deep Listening, 5
"Too-tight clothes," 78–81, 86
Transcendental Meditation, 12
Tree Pose, 93, **94**, 95, 248, **248**

V

Visualization
Elevator to a Welcoming Arrival,
17–19, 26
Hourglass Mediation, 39
in metta meditation, 195–99
Vulnerability, 111

W

Walk, mindful, 53
Welcome, 15–26
message, 16
practices for welcoming ourselves,
17–26
Contemplation, 17
Instant Pause and Reset, 26
Journaling Prompt, 25
Meditation Experience, 18–19
Relaxmore, 24
Restorative Yoga Experience,
22–23, **23**
Yoga Experience, 20, **21**

Well-being, 212–13
being here, 54
cultivating by relaxing into the life we
have right now, 14
description of, 13–14, 232
future, 230
habits/feelings that lessen, 114, 166,
223
intention and, 216
nurtured by relaxation, 232
Wisdom center, 154, 182, 212
Wolf (Native American tale), 210

Y

Yoga
Deep Listening Yoga Sequence,
234–58
mindful yoga practice, 157–58
in sample weekly practice schedule, 9
Yoga blankets, 8–9, 264–66, **265-66**
Yoga blocks, 8, 264, 267, **267**
Yoga Experience
Cat/Cow Flow, 68–69, **68-69**
Child's Pose, 226, **227**
Flowing Warrior 2, **169**, 169–72, **171**
Gecko Arm Flowing Cobra, 144–45,
144-45
Hero Pose, 20, **21**
Low Lunge, 200–201, **201**
Mountain Chair Flow, 42, **43**
Mountain Pose, **40**, 41
Standing Flowing Twist, 119, **120-21**
Tree Pose, 93, **94**, 95
Yoga strap, 9, 264

CREDITS

Mats by Priti Yoga

page 28 *Excerpt reprinted from Tara Brach. *True Refuge.*
New York: Bantam Books, 2012.